Rapid Review Anesthesiology Oral Boards

Rapid Review Anesthesiology Oral Boards

Edited by

Ruchir Gupta, MD

Assistant Professor of Anesthesiology,
North Shore University-Hofstra Medical School,
Dix Hills, NY, USA

Associate editor

Minh Chau Joseph Tran, MD

Assistant Professor of Anesthesiology,
UMDNJ-New Jersey Medical School,
Department of Anesthesiology, Newark, NJ, USA

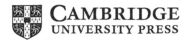

CAMBRIDGE
UNIVERSITY PRESS

CAMBRIDGE
UNIVERSITY PRESS

University Printing House, Cambridge CB2 8BS, United Kingdom

Cambridge University Press is part of the University of Cambridge.

It furthers the University's mission by disseminating knowledge in the pursuit of education, learning and research at the highest international levels of excellence.

www.cambridge.org
Information on this title: www.cambridge.org/9781107653665

© Cambridge University Press 2013

First published 2013

A catalogue record for this publication is available from the British Library

Library of Congress Cataloguing in Publication data
Rapid review anesthesiology oral boards / edited by Ruchir Gupta ; associate editor, Minh Chau Joseph Tran
   p. ; cm.
Includes bibliographical references and index.
ISBN 978-1-107-65366-5 (pbk.)
I. Gupta, Ruchir, editor of compilation.   II. Tran, Minh Chau Joseph, editor of compilation.
[DNLM: 1. Anesthesiology–methods–Examination Questions.   2. Anesthesia–Examination Questions.   3. Anesthetics–Examination Questions. WO 218.2]
RD82.3
617.9'6076–dc23
2013020827

ISBN 978-1-107-65366-5 Paperback

Contents

Section 3: Orthopedics

Section 4: Trauma

Section 5: Urology

Section 6: Pediatrics

Contributors

Xiaodong Bao
Staff Anesthesiologist, Emcare Anesthesiology, Dallas, TX, USA

Edouard Belotte
Staff Anesthesiologist, North American Partners in Anesthesia, USA

Monique Cadogan
Assistant Professor of Anesthesiology, New York Medical College, Westchester Medical Center, Valhalla, NY, USA

John Cooley
Attending Anesthesiologist, Westchester Medical Center, Valhalla, NY, USA

Shimon Frankel
Staff Anesthesiologist, North Shore University Hospital, Manhasset, NY, USA

Sheryl Glassman
Resident, Department of Anesthesiology and Perioperative Medicine, Drexel University College of Medicine, Philadelphia, PA, USA

Anita Gupta
Associate Professor of Anesthesiology and Perioperative Medicine, Drexel University College of Medicine, Philadelphia, PA, USA

Ruchir Gupta
Assistant Professor of Anesthesiology, Hofstra North Shore-LIJ School of Medicine, Hempstead, NY, USA

Aimee Gretchen Kakascik
Assistant Professor, Department of Anesthesiology and Pediatrics, Baylor College of Medicine, Texas Children's Hospital, Houston, TX, USA

Sarah J. Madison
Assistant Clinical Professor, Department of Anesthesiology, University of California, San Diego, CA, USA

Joseph Marino
Director of Anesthesia, North Shore LIJ at Franklin Hospital, Valley Stream, NY, USA

Julio R. Olaya
Assistant Professor of Anesthesiology and Critical Care, SLU School of Medicine, and Pediatric Anesthesiologist at Cardinal Glennon Children's Medical Center, St. Louis, MO, USA

Federico Osorio
Cardiothoracic Anesthesiologist, Anesthesia Consultants of Dallas, and Creative Director – Founder, MD Cloud Solutions, Dallas, TX, USA

Raymond Pesso
Chairman, Department of Anesthesiology, Medical Director, Perioperative Services, Nassau University Medical Center; Assistant Professor of Clinical Anesthesiology, Hofstra North Shore-LIJ School of Medicine, Hempstead, NY, USA

Sergey V. Pisklakov
Assistant Professor, Department of Anesthesiology, University of Medicine and Dentistry of New Jersey – New Jersey Medical School, Newark, NJ, USA

Mark Slomovits
Attending Anesthesiologist, North Shore University Hospital, Manhasset, NY, USA

Jaspreet Singh Toor
New York College of Osteopathic Medicine, NY, USA

Barbara Vickers
Attending Anesthesiologist, North Shore-LIJ Hospital, Valley Stream, NY, USA

Nicholas Weber
Resident, Department of Anesthesiology and Perioperative Medicine, Drexel University College of Medicine, Philadelphia, PA, USA

Peggy Wingard
Assistant Professor, University of Texas Medical Branch, Galveston, TX, USA

Stanley Yuan
Resident Anesthesiologist, New York Medical College, Westchester Medical Center, Valhalla, NY, USA

Abbreviations

AAA	abdominal aortic aneurysm
ABG	arterial blood gas
ACC/AHA	American College of Cardiology/American Heart Association
ACT	activated clotting time
ADH	antidiuretic hormone
aDP	aortic diastolic pressure
ADP	adenosine diphosphate
AFOI	awake fiberoptic intubation
AICD	automatic internal cardiac defibrillator
APUD	amine precursor uptake and decarboxylation
ARDS	acute respiratory distress syndrome
AS	aortic stenosis
ASA	American Society of Anesthesiologists; aspirin
ASD	atrial septal defect
ASRA	American Society of Regional Anesthesia and Pain Medicine
AVM	arteriovenous malformation
BE	base excess
BID	twice daily dosing
BMI	body mass index
BMP	basic metabolic panel
BP	blood pressure
bpm	beats per minute
BSA	body surface area
BUN	blood urea nitrogen
CABG	coronary artery bypass graft
CAD	coronary artery disease
CBC	complete blood count
CBF	cerebral blood flow
CBV	cerebral blood volume
CDH	congenital diaphragmatic hernia
CF	cystic fibrosis
CHD	congenital heart disease
CHF	congestive heart failure

CI	cardiac index
$CMRO_2$	cerebral oxygen metabolic rate
CMV	controlled mandatory ventilation
CNS	central nervous system
CO	carbon monoxide; cardiac output
CO_2	carbon dioxide
COPD	chronic obstructive pulmonary disease
CPAP	continuous positive airway pressure
CPB	cardiopulmonary bypass
CPP	cerebral perfusion pressure
CPR	cardiopulmonary resuscitation
Cr	creatinine
CRF	chronic renal failure
CRPS	chronic regional pain syndrome
CSF	cerebrospinal fluid
CSWS	cerebral salt wasting syndrome
CT	computed tomography
CTA	clear to auscultation
CV	cardiovascular
CVP	central venous catheter
CXR	chest X-ray
DBP	diastolic blood pressure
DDAVP	desmopressin
DIC	disseminated intravascular coagulation
DLT	double lumen tube
DM	diabetes mellitus
2,3-DPG	2,3-diphosphoglycerate
DVT	deep venous thrombosis
ECMO	extracorporeal membrane oxygenation
ED_{95}	effective dose in 95% of patients
EF	ejection fraction
EKG	electrocardiogram
EMG	electromyography
ENT	ear nose throat
ER	emergency room
ESR	erythrocyte sedimentation rate
ESRD	end-stage renal disease
$ETCO_2$	end-tidal carbon dioxide
ETT	endotracheal tube
FAST	focused assessment with sonography for trauma
FeNA	fractional excretion of sodium
FFP	fresh frozen plasma
FHR	fetal heart rate
FiO_2	fraction of inspired oxygen

FOI	fiberoptic intubation
FRC	functional residual capacity
FVL	flow volume loop
g	gauge; gram
G6P	glucose 6-phosphate
GA	general anesthesia
GABA	gamma-aminobutyric acid
GCS	Glasgow Coma Scale
GERD	gastroesophageal reflux disease
GI	gastrointestinal
GMP	guanosine monophosphate
GU	genitourinary
H&P	history and physical
H/H	hemoglobin/hematocrit
Hb	hemoglobin
HbA	hemoglobin A
Hct	hematocrit
HCTZ	hydrochlorothiazide
HD	hemodynamic
HELLP	hemolytic anemia, elevated liver enzymes, low platelets
HFOV	high-frequency oscillatory ventilation
HLA	human leukocyte antigen
HOCM	hypertrophic cardiomyopathy
HPI	history of present illness
HPV	hypoxic pulmonary vasoconstriction
HR	heart rate
5HT3	serotonin
HTN	hypertension
I&D	incision and drainage
IABP	intra-aortic balloon pump
IBW	ideal body weight
ICP	intracranial pressure
ICU	intensive care unit
IE	infective endocarditis
IUGR	intrauterine growth retardation
IV	intravenous
IVC	inferior vena cava
IVDA	intravenous drug abuse
IVH	intraventricular hemorrhage
IVIG	intravenous immunoglobulin
JVD	jugular venous distention
K	potassium
LMA	laryngeal mask airway
LMWH	low molecular weight heparin

LR	lactated Ringer's
LUQ	left upper quadrant
LVEDP	left ventricular end-diastolic pressure
LVEF	left ventricular ejection fraction
LVH	left ventricular hypertrophy
MA	maximum amplitude
MAC	mean alveolar concentration
MAP	mean arterial pressure
METs	metabolic equivalent
MG	myasthenia gravis
MH	malignant hyperthermia
MI	myocardial infarction
MRI	magnetic resonance imaging
MS	mitral stenosis
Na	sodium
NAS	neonatal abstinence syndrome
NC	nasal cannula
NDMR	nondepolarizing muscle relaxant
NEC	necrotizing enterocolitis
NG	nasogastric
NGT	nasogastric tube
NIBP	non-invasive BP cuff
NICU	neonatal intensive care unit
NIF	negative inspiratory force
NKDA	no known drug allergy
NPO	nil per os
NS	normal saline
NSAID	nonsteroidal anti-inflammatory drug
NSR	normal sinus rhythm
OG	orogastric
OLV	one lung ventilation
OPCAB	off-pump coronary artery bypass
OR	operating room
ORIF	open reduction internal fixation
OSA	obstructive sleep apnea
OSH	obstructive sleep hypopnea
P	pulse; pressure
$P(A\text{-}a)O_2$	alveolar-arterial oxygen pressure gradient
PA	pulmonary artery
PAC	pulmonary artery catheter
$PaCO_2$	partial pressure of carbon dioxide, arterial
PACU	post anesthesia care unit
PaO_2	partial pressure of oxygen, arterial
PAP	peak airway pressure

PCA	patient-controlled analgesia
PCEA	patient-controlled epidural analgesia
PCWP	pulmonary capillary wedge pressure
PDA	patent ductus arteriosus
PDHD	post-dural puncture headache
PE	physical examination; pulmonary embolism
PEEP	positive end-expiratory pressure
PFO	patent foramen ovale
PFT	pulmonary function test
PICU	pediatric intensive care unit
PIH	pregnancy-induced hypertension
PIV	peripheral intravenous
Plt	platelets
PMH	past medical history
PO	per os (per mouth)
POCD	postoperative cognitive dysfunction
POD	postoperative day
PPH	postpartum hemorrhage
PRBC	packed red blood cells
PS	Pickwickian syndrome
PSH	past surgical history
PTX	pneumothorax
PVC	premature ventricular contractions
PVR	pulmonary vascular resistance
QD	per day
R → L	right to left
RA	room air
RAP	right atrial pressure
RBC	red blood cell
RBF	renal blood flow
RLN	recurrent laryngeal nerve
ROM	range of motion
RRR	regular rate and rhythm
RSI	rapid sequence induction
RUL	right upper lobe
RUQ	right upper quadrant
SAH	subarachnoid hemorrhage
SAM	systolic anterior motion
SaO_2	oxygen saturation
SBP	systolic blood pressure
SCD	sickle cell disease
SCPP	spinal cord perfusion pressure
SH	smoking history
SIADH	syndrome of inappropriate antidiuretic hormone secretion

SICU	surgical intensive care unit
SIMV	synchronized intermittent mandatory ventilation
SLT	single lumen tube
SSEP	somatosensory evoked potential
STAT	immediate(ly)
SVC	superior vena cava
SVR	systemic vascular resistance
SVT	supraventricular tachycardia
T	temperature
T_3	triiodothyronine
T_4	thyroxine
TEE	transesophageal echocardiogram
TEF	tracheoesophageal fistula
TEG	thromboelastogram
TENS	transcutaneous electrical nerve stimulation
TIVA	total intravenous anesthesia
TPN	total parenteral nutrition
TRALI	transfusion-related lung injury
TURP	transurethral resection of prostate
UA	urinalysis
UO	urinary output
V/Q	ventilation/perfusion
VAE	venous air embolism
VATS	video-assisted thoracic surgery
VMA	vanillylmandelic acid
VS	vital signs
VSD	ventricular septal defect
VVBP	venovenous bypass
vWD	von Willebrand's disease
vWF	von Willebrand factor
WBC	white blood cell
WHO	World Health Organization

Introduction

The anesthesia board exam in most parts of the world is typically divided into two parts: a written multiple choice exam and an oral exam in which a clinical scenario, or "stem," is presented and questions are asked by the examiner related to this stem.

In the US, you will have two sessions: a Part 1 session with a long stem in which you will be asked questions regarding the intraoperative and postoperative care and a Part 2 session where you will be given a slightly shorter stem and be asked preoperative and intraoperative questions. You will have a short amount of time to review and "dissect" your stem before entering the examination room. Upon entering, there will be two individuals sitting behind a desk who will be asking the questions. At the end of each stem you are given three short "additional topics" scenarios and 4–5 questions per scenario. These additional topics are often harder than your main stems because you have no time to review and "dissect" the clinical scenario and the questions they ask can be preoperative, intraoperative, or postoperative.

How to approach the oral boards

The oral boards were not created merely to test knowledge. Successful completion of the written exam attests to the fact you have sufficient knowledge. Rather, it is meant to determine if you can adequately discuss anesthesia as a trained consultant. The Board wants you to describe everything you do. For example, if asked how you would induce an ASA 1 patient for a cholecystectomy, you cannot say "propofol." You must begin by saying, "After preoxygenating with 100% O_2, and ensuring the airway is normal, I will administer fentanyl, lidocaine, propofol, and after ensuring that I can ventilate, rocuronium."

If the philosophy of the entire exam could be summed up in one word, it would be "why." What you do is not as important as why you do it, so you must give an explanation for your decision. In doing so, it is advisable that you use the term "risks outweighing benefits" or vice versa. Consider the following example:

Question: Would you administer propofol to a patient with severe CAD?

Answer: "No I would not because the risks of propofol administration in a patient with severe CAD outweigh the benefits. Propofol is a fast-acting drug that can provide rapid intubating conditions. However, it is associated with hypotension, which can decrease the coronary perfusion pressure necessary to perfuse the myocardium. Thus, I would rather choose a more cardiac stable drug such as etomidate."

Such an answer allows the examiner to follow your thought process and also determine your level of knowledge. Mostly all decisions in anesthesia have a risk/benefit ratio and discussing this ratio in your answer will impress your examiners.

Not a comprehensive review

This exam is not a spectator sport; it's a tackle sport. Neither this book, nor any on this topic can, by itself, get you ready for the exam. You must do practice exams! At our course, www.justoralboards.com, we offer practice mock oral exams that provide similar conditions as the actual test. Once in the "hot seat" candidates often find their knowledge disappearing within the shroud of anxiety and nervousness. They also find it difficult to organize their thoughts. This book can help you understand how to formulate your answers and which subtopics to keep in mind when you see your stem, but it cannot, by itself, relieve your anxiety or help you organize your thoughts. For this, you must practice, practice, practice!

How to use this book

The examiners have certain topics they love. Within each topic are "subtopics" that they will inevitably question you on. For example, if your stem is about a patient undergoing a pulmonary lobectomy, you can be certain that the questions they will ask will be about double lumen tube (DLT) indications/contraindications, diagnosis of accurate placement of DLT, management of hypoxia after placement of DLT, etc. Knowing what the questions will likely be prior to entering your exam room allows you to formulate your responses and be ready for the questions as they arrive.

Thus, this book is organized into individual chapters of the 34 high yield exam topics seen on the anesthesia boards. In addition, there are 5 additional chapters that each contain 10 "additional topics" based on subspecialty. Within each of the 32 high yield exam topics are the most common subtopics that are tested, and a few questions are provided modeled around the subtopics. Most likely if you have a stem on one of these 32 topics you will also have questions similar to the ones in the chapter for that topic. Read it! Look at how the answer is formulated! Then, team up with a study partner and test each other using the stems provided to you.

Often times candidates will want to practice mock oral exams but they lack full length exams with questions AND answers that they can trust to use in testing one another. This book is a solution to that. We encourage the "study-buddy" system and, because this book is pocket size, you can carry it around with you during your clinical day and review any exam on your own during your down time.

Learn the language

As you review for this test, you will realize that this exam has its own unique language. The examiners want you to speak a certain way, using certain terms. As you review the chapters, you will realize how different this language is from the one you speak every day. Many candidates fail every year not for the lack of knowledge, but because they didn't appreciate the jargon and terminology that the anesthesia boards desire. By providing you with answers, this book hopes you will learn the language and use it as you move forward with your study.

Format

Each chapter in this book has been written in either the Stem 1 (long form) or Stem 2 (short form) format. Our desire in doing so was to give you the opportunity to practice "dissecting" both types of stems. In the exam, Stem 1 questions will be strictly in the intraoperative and postoperative areas whereas Stem 2 questions will be preoperative and intraoperative. For your benefit, we have provided questions on preoperative, intraoperative, and postoperative sections for all of the stems, regardless of whether or not they were 1 or 2. This way, you will be familiar with the major subtopics in each facet of anesthesia care.

Also, the level of difficulty in each exam has purposely been kept at a slightly lower level than the exams you would normally encounter with our course, www. justoralboards.com. This is intentional. We want you to first develop a solid, broad-based foundation by learning about the major high yield topics for the oral exam. Once you have mastered these 34 high yield topics, you will be in a good position to start taking more difficult exams, in which multiple topics are combined. For example, perhaps the patient having a pulmonary lobectomy has sickle cell disease. In this book, these topics are covered separately, but once you understand the anesthetic implications of both and what key subtopics the examiner would want to cover in each of these, you are in a better position to begin integrating these concepts.

Finally, have faith in yourself and your abilities as a clinician. If you are studying for the oral exam, you already have a great deal to be proud of. You obviously have a solid knowledge base (which you perhaps forgot by now but can easily relearn) and you completed an anesthesia residency. Thus, you know how to administer anesthesia. Use this book to review what you have already done and speak to your examiner like you are speaking to a third year medical student, leaving out no details and being thorough in your response and explanation. Work hard, study hard, and do as many mock orals as you can. Every time you are about to give up, just think how much better you will feel when you click on your exam score and see the word "PASS." Take it from two people who did it the first time around, it's worth all the agony and heartache.

Obesity/difficult airway

Ruchir Gupta

STEM 1

A 38 year old, 190 kg 5′6″ male is scheduled for a laparoscopic gastric bypass.

PMH: Patient has DM, HTN, GERD, OSA requiring CPAP. His past medical history is also significant for hypertension, severe GERD, hiatal hernia, depression, and obstructive sleep apnea requiring CPAP.

PE: P 74 bpm, BP 130/68 mmHg, RR 14, T 36°C, 97% on room air. On physical exam, his Mallampati score is III and his cervical range of motion is normal. His dentition is intact. Auscultation reveals normal breath sounds bilaterally with regular rate and rhythm.

EKG: NSR.

Labs: Serum glucose is 153 mg/dL, otherwise his complete blood count (CBC) and basic chemistry panel are within normal limits.

Preoperative

Obesity

1. **How is body mass index (BMI) calculated?**
   BMI is calculated by dividing the weight in kg by the height in meters squared (kg/m^2).

Rapid Review Anesthesiology Oral Boards, ed. Ruchir Gupta and Minh Chau Joseph Tran. Published by Cambridge University Press. © Cambridge University Press 2013.

Obstructive sleep apnea

2. **How is obstructive sleep apnea (OSA) different from obstructive sleep hypopnea (OSH)?**

   OSA is cessation of airflow for >10 seconds, five or more times per hour of sleep. There is a >4% decrease in O_2 while the patient is asleep. By contrast, in obstructive sleep hypopnea (OSH) there is a decrease in airflow of >50% for more than 10 seconds, 15 or more times per hour of sleep. The decrease in O_2 saturation during these episodes is also >4%.

3. **How is the definitive diagnosis of OSA made?**

   Although OSA may be suspected by history, physical examination, and/ or comorbidities, a definitive diagnosis requires a formal sleep study.

4. **What are the systemic manifestations of OSA?**

   OSA affects multiple organ systems:

   Cardiac – patients usually have hypertension and LVH. Pulmonary HTN may also be present.

   Pulmonary – increased V/Q mismatch from decreased FRC and atelectasis.

   GI – patients often have the stomach displaced upward due to extra-abdominal pressure placing them at risk for GERD.

   Renal – the patient may have hypertensive nephropathy.

   Neuro – hypersomnolence is frequently observed with increased sensitivity to anesthetic agents.

5. **How is OSA distinguished from the Pickwickian syndrome?**

   OSA is defined as cessation of airflow for >10 seconds, five or more times per hour of sleep. Pickwickian syndrome (PS) is characterized by chronic hypoventilation which is worse during sleep, resulting in an elevation in $PaCO_2$ levels. Indeed, the diagnosis of PS is BMI >30, $PaCO_2$ >44 mmHg and no alternate explanation for hypoventilation. Patients with PS often have coexisting OSA, but not every patient with one disease will necessarily have the other. Patients with PS frequently develop sequelae from the CO_2 retention: polycythemia, cor pulmonale, and somnolence.

6. **How does this patient's history of OSA affect your anesthetic management?**

   Preoperatively, a thorough H&P must be done to assess for any comorbid conditions. I would use sedative drugs cautiously because of increased sensitivity in OSA patients to CNS depressants such as midazolam. A thorough airway exam must also be done because most of these patients are difficult airways. Intraoperatively, care must be taken to preoxygenate these patients thoroughly as they are prone to rapid desaturation secondary to low FRC. I would also have the difficult airway cart in the room and consider an awake intubation if the airway was nonreassuring. During the course of the surgery, I would use a multimodal pain management regimen including IV NSAIDs, IV Tylenol, rectus sheath block, and local wound infiltration to decrease my narcotic use. Postoperatively, I will extubate in the head-up position to improve pulmonary mechanics and extubate only after the patient is fully awake. I will also have a CPAP machine ready in the PACU and continue to monitor the patient closely in the PACU for any episodes of apnea and desaturation.

Intraoperative

Monitors

1. **What monitors will you use for this patient?**
   I would use the standard ASA monitors (pulse oximeter, noninvasive blood pressure measurements, a five-lead EKG, a temperature probe, and a capnograph), a neuromuscular blockade monitor, and if PIV access is difficult, I will place a central line. I will also ask for a Foley catheter to be placed.

2. **The nurse informs you that she has a large size BP cuff. What will you do?**
   I could attempt to place a standard size BP cuff on the forearm or the lower leg. I could also place a large size cuff or alternatively, an arterial line.

Premedication

3. **What premedication if any will you give this patient?**
   To avoid possible respiratory depression in morbidly obese patients with OSA, premedication is used sparingly, if at all. Thus, if the patient was anxious, I would start by reassuring the patient. If the patient was still anxious, then after monitors have been placed in the operating room, I would administer a low dose of midazolam and/or ketamine. Due to risk of aspiration, I would administer sodium citrate to decrease stomach acidity, and promotility agents such as metoclopramide to enhance gastric emptying.

Intubation

4. **How would you intubate this patient?**
   Based on information provided, management of the patient's airway may be difficult and so after preoxygenating the patient with 100% oxygen, I would perform an awake oral fiberoptic intubation. I would topicalize the airway with 1–2% lidocaine spray or nebulizer and perform a superior laryngeal nerve block by injecting 2 mL of 2% lidocaine, just anterior to the cornu of the hyoid bones, and a transtracheal recurrent laryngeal nerve block.

5. **Your resident accidentally administers a bolus of propofol to the patient to prevent him from moving during the AFOI. A few seconds later, the patient becomes apneic and begins to desaturate. What will you do?**
   I will immediately call for help and perform mask ventilation in an attempt to improve this patient's oxygenation while attempting to awaken the patient.

6. **You mask ventilate the patient and obtain some EtCO$_2$, but the patient continues to desaturate, with an oxygen saturation of 90% and decreasing. Mask ventilation is getting progressively more difficult. What will you do?**
   I will again call for help if it has not yet arrived and perform direct laryngoscopy. If that did not work or I am unable to mask ventilate the patient, I would place an LMA and ventilate through that device.

7. **You successfully place an LMA and the desaturation improves. Should you cancel the case once the patient awakens?**
   It depends on the status of the patient. If there is a great deal of oral swelling and bleeding secondary to my ventilation and direct laryngoscopy attempts, I would delay this case for a few days until the swelling has subsided. If, however, the oropharynx seemed uninjured and there were no signs of bleeding or swelling, I would reattempt my awake fiberoptic and proceed as scheduled.

Maintenance of anesthesia

8. **The airway is now secured with an ETT. What agents will you use to maintain anesthesia?**
   I would choose short-acting agents to reduce the risk of postoperative sedation. Desflurane is desirable because it is relatively insoluble in fat, has a fast wake-up, faster return of airway reflexes, and decreased amount of hepatic metabolism. For muscle relaxation, I will choose cisatracurium or rocuronium.

Postoperative

Extubation

1. **Would you extubate this patient? If so, how?**
   Assuming there were no adverse intraoperative events and significant volume shifts, then I would want to extubate this patient immediately at the end of the procedure. I would have emergency airway equipment on standby, place the patient in the sitting position to optimize pulmonary mechanics, ensure the patient has been adequately reversed, and have the patient spontaneously breathing with adequate tidal volumes and a normal respiratory rate. Once the patient is responding to commands and able to protect his airway, I will extubate.

2. **What respiratory parameters can be used for extubation?**
   Respiratory rates between 10 and 30 breaths per minute, SaO$_2$ greater than 95% on FiO$_2$ of 0.4, vital capacity greater than 10 mL/kg of IBW, and tidal volume greater than 5 mL/kg of IBW.

Hyperglycemia

3. **The nurse in the PACU pages you to tell you the patient's blood glucose is 253 mg/dL. Why is controlling blood glucose in the perioperative period important?**
   The consequences of acute hyperglycemia include impaired immune response with increased risk of infection, impaired wound healing, dehydration, and electrolyte disturbances secondary to the osmotic diuretic effect of high serum glucose levels. This diabetic patient, who takes oral hypoglycemic medication, is at risk for developing potentially fatal nonketotic hyperosmolar coma.

Pain control

4. **What is your plan for postoperative pain management in this patient?**
   I would provide this patient with non-opioid analgesics such as Tylenol and NSAIDs. I would also have asked the surgeon to place local anesthesia around the incisions intraoperatively. In addition, for pain refractory to these medications, a patient-controlled analgesia (PCA) is helpful in providing relief without risking overdosing since the patient must be awake and alert to administer the medicine. Due to the presence of OSA I would place this patient in a monitored setting overnight.

5. **A colleague suggests the use of patient-controlled epidural analgesia (PCEA), instead of PCA. What are some benefits of PCEA, in comparison to PCA?**
   The benefit of PCEA over PCA is that less opioid medication is used because local anesthesia can also be delivered epidurally. The lower opioid requirement results in fewer side effects such as respiratory complications while also ensuring effective analgesia.

Mental status change

6. **A few hours later, the PACU nurse informs you that the patient is "disoriented." What is your differential diagnosis?**
   My differential includes:
   (1) Unstable vital signs: hypoxia, hypotension, malignant arrhythmia.
   (2) Anesthesia-induced causes: residual anesthesia, narcotic overdose or reaction.
   (3) Possible delirium tremens from withdrawal from a previously unknown substance abuse agent.
   (4) Potential metabolic and endocrinologic causes: hyponatremia, hypokalemia, hypocalcemia, hypoglycemia, hyperglycemia, hypothermia, hypothyroidism, and Addison's disease, among others.
   (5) Neurologic causes include post-ictal state, cerebral edema, and stroke.

7. **How will you respond?**
   First, I will ensure that the patient is adequately oxygenating and ventilating and the vital signs are stable. Next, I will perform a focused history and physical.

From the history, I will review the anesthetic record as well as the nurse's notes to see what medications the patient has received, when the symptoms began, have they been getting worse or better, and the severity of the disorientation. From the physical, I will listen for breath sounds and look for neurologic signs, including pupillary size and any focal neurologic deficits. Finally, I will order STAT labs including ABG, electrolytes with glucose, and a CBC to evaluate for anemia. If a stroke is suspected, a STAT head CT and neurology consult would be obtained.

FURTHER READING

Barash P. G., Cullen B. F., Stoelting R. K., Cahalan M., Stock C. M. (eds.). *Clinical Anesthesia*, 6th edn. Philadelphia, PA: Lippincott Williams & Wilkins, 2009.

Miller R. D., Eriksson L. I., Fleisher L. A., Wiener-Kornish J. P., Young W. L. (eds.). *Miller's Anesthesia*, 7th edn. Philadelphia, PA: Churchill Livingstone Elsevier, 2010.

Yao F., Fontes M. L., Malhotra V. (eds.). *Yao and Artusio's Anesthesiology: Problem-Oriented Patient Management*, 7th edn. Philadelphia, PA: Lippincott Williams & Wilkins, 2011.

2

Myasthenia gravis

Shimon Frankel

STEM 2

A 54 year old female presents for laparoscopic resection of the colon. Patient has a history of colon cancer and myasthenia gravis for which she is on pyridostigmine and prednisone. VS: BP 121/55 mmHg, RR 12, HR 64 bpm, room air saturation 99%. Hb 11.4 g/dL.

Preoperative

Assessment of severity

1. **How would you assess if this patient is optimized for surgery?**
   I would obtain a focused history and physical. From the history, I want to know if her disease is limited to ocular muscles, or if there is involvement of her extremities or respiratory/laryngeal muscles as evidenced by trouble chewing, swallowing, or talking. I would also want to know if the patient ever had surgery before, any prolonged intubations or problems with anesthesia, any episodes of myasthenic crisis, and whether her symptoms have been stable over the past few weeks. From the physical, I would assess bilateral motor strength in all of her extremities, and see if she displays any signs of pharyngeal or respiratory muscle involvement.

2. **What is myasthenia gravis (MG)? What other medical conditions is MG closely associated with?**
   MG is an autoimmune disorder involving antibodies to the alpha-subunit of the postsynaptic nicotinic acetylcholine receptor at the neuromuscular junction leading to a decreased number of functional receptors. With repeated

Rapid Review Anesthesiology Oral Boards, ed. Ruchir Gupta and Minh Chau Joseph Tran. Published by Cambridge University Press. © Cambridge University Press 2013.

stimulation and decreased acetylcholine release, fatigue occurs. The extent of involvement can be limited to ocular muscles, but muscles of respiration and swallowing can also be involved, causing respiratory distress or aspiration.

MG is occasionally associated with thymus hyperplasia, thymomas, or autoimmune diseases such as thyroid disease, pernicious anemia, rheumatoid arthritis, and women with certain HLA types.

3. **Would you obtain pulmonary function tests (PFTs)? Why? Why not?**
   I would not obtain PFTs in this patient unless there was a severe respiratory component as evidenced by my H&P. If the patient had severe respiratory symptoms, negative inspiratory force (NIF) and forced vital capacity (FVC) could be used as a reference to determine optimal conditions for extubation or the need for postoperative mechanical ventilation. They may also help in determining appropriateness for ambulatory surgery. If the patient has a thymoma, flow volume loops (FVLs) can demonstrate the extent of impairment and whether it is fixed or dynamic.

Medication for MG

4. **Should the patient continue the morning dose of pyridostigmine on the day of surgery? Why?**
   Although there is no clear-cut answer, I would recommend continuing the pyridostigmine in order to avoid any possible respiratory difficulties prior to surgery. The disadvantage of continuing cholinesterase inhibition is the possibility of prolonged motor block with succinylcholine, and the possibility of developing a cholinergic crisis.

5. **Why is this patient on corticosteroids?**
   MG is an autoimmune disease. Corticosteroids suppress the immune system and attenuate the production of these abnormal autoantibodies to the acetylcholine receptors at the motor endplate. Treatment of MG usually begins with cholinesterase inhibitors. For more advanced disease, corticosteroids and thymectomy are used. In more severe cases, immunosuppressants (such as azathioprine or cyclosporine) and plasmapheresis are used. IVIG is used for myasthenic crisis.

6. **Would you administer preoperative steroids? Why? Why not?**
   Yes, I would administer a stress dose of steroids, hydrocortisone 100 mg every 8 hours on the day of surgery and then taper it postoperatively. Patients taking chronic glucocorticoids may have suppressed adrenal function. Thus I would continue her chronic dose perioperatively and be alert for signs of adrenal insufficiency.

7. **Would you sedate this patient preoperatively?**
   If there is a question as to her respiratory reserve I would avoid sedative premedication. If the symptoms are primarily ocular, a small dose of a

benzodiazepine would be acceptable, especially since emotional stress could exacerbate myasthenia.

8. **Is there anything you would tell this patient about her postoperative course?**
I would inform the patient and family that symptoms may worsen perioperatively, but will usually return to baseline. I would also mention the possibility of postoperative mechanical ventilation.

Lambert–Eaton syndrome

9. **What is Lambert–Eaton myasthenic syndrome (LEMS)?**
This is a disease of motor weakness that is often characterized by proximal limb weakness, especially of the lower extremities. It is caused by autoantibodies to the voltage-gated calcium channels of the presynaptic membrane. Calcium is not able to enter the nerve ending and allow acetylcholine release. Weakness typically improves with repetitive use as this enables buildup of calcium allowing for acetylcholine release. Patients are sensitive to both depolarizing and nondepolarizing muscle relaxants and patients may need postoperative respiratory support.

LEMS is often seen as a paraneoplastic syndrome related to small cell cancer of the lung. It may also be seen with sarcoidosis, other malignancies, thyroiditis, and collagen vascular diseases.

Intraoperative

Anesthesia

1. **Would you select a general or a regional technique for this patient?**
Assuming there are no contraindications, I would prefer a regional anesthetic technique for this case because it avoids muscle relaxation, instrumenting of the airway, and the need for postoperative ventilator support. Patients with MG are usually more resistant to succinylcholine and more sensitive to nondepolarizing muscle relaxants.

2. **If you decide on a regional technique, would you select a spinal or an epidural approach?**
I would select a continuous epidural approach because it would allow me to run a constant infusion if the operation takes longer than was originally planned. Additionally, it allows me to administer local anesthetics and narcotics postoperatively for pain.

Induction

3. **How will you induce general anesthesia in this patient if she refuses a regional technique?**

   Assuming the patient has a normal airway, I will preoxygenate with 100% oxygen and perform a slow controlled induction with short-acting agents such as remifentanil, lidocaine, and propofol.

4. **The surgeon says he will need muscle relaxation for the case. How do you respond?**

   I would try to avoid muscle relaxants if possible because even patients with minimal disease may have increased sensitivity to NDMR. Additionally, inhalational agents often provide adequate muscle relaxation in myasthenic patients to perform surgery. If needed, I would use intermediate-acting muscle relaxants in increments of 0.1–0.2 times the ED_{95}.

5. **How would your induction technique change if the patient were at high risk of aspiration?**

   I would perform a rapid sequence intubation using succinylcholine at a dose of 1.5–2 mg/kg. Patients with MG are resistant to succinylcholine, but at higher doses it should provide rapid intubating conditions.

Muscle relaxation

6. **Would you use a nerve stimulator during the case? Why? Why not?**

   Yes I would but I would bear in mind that it may not be reliable in myasthenic patients because the distribution of muscle weakness is often uneven and many patients may exhibit fade even in the preoperative period.

7. **What is the impact of preoperative cholinesterase inhibitor administration on neuromuscular blockade and reversal?**

   Preoperative pyridostigmine inhibits plasma cholinesterase and succinylcholine may cause a prolonged block. Reversal of residual nondepolarizing neuromuscular blockade at the end of surgery may be unsuccessful because acetylcholinesterase is already maximally inhibited.

Postoperative

Postoperative weakness

1. **Are you going to extubate this patient at the end of the case?**

   It depends on how the case went and whether the patient is meeting extubation criteria. I would not extubate if more than minimal doses of nondepolarizing muscle blocking agents or narcotics were used since the patient may not recover respiratory function immediately.

2. **You receive a call from the PACU complaining that the patient is feeling weak. What do you think? What will you do?**

Many factors could cause postoperative weakness in a patient with myasthenia gravis. My differentials would include residual muscle relaxant, narcotic overdose, residual inhalational anesthetic, myasthenic crisis, cholinergic crisis, hypothermia, hypocarbia, and acidosis.

I would assess the patient's vital signs, saturation, and respiratory pattern. If the patient was showing signs of respiratory insufficiency, I would reintubate her. If she were stable, I would look for the cause of her weakness, review the anesthetic record, and consider a Tensilon (edrophonium) test to evaluate if she was in myasthenic crisis rather than cholinergic crisis. With myasthenic crisis her symptoms should improve with edrophonium; with cholinergic crisis, they would not.

Crisis

3. **What is a myasthenic crisis? What are the precipitating factors?**

A myasthenic crisis, which implies severe bulbar or respiratory symptoms, can be precipitated by progression of disease or other factors. Some factors that may worsen symptoms are infection, recent surgery, emotional stress, and interruption of immunosuppressants. Drugs associated with worsening symptoms include aminoglycosides, polymyxins, fluoroquinolones, clindamycin, anticonvulsants, beta blockers, calcium channel blockers, corticosteroids, local anesthetics, magnesium, ketamine, neuromuscular blockers, and anticholinergics. Hypothermia, acidosis, and electrolyte abnormalities such as hypokalemia or hypermagnesemia can compound the severe muscle weakness.

4. **What is a cholinergic crisis? How would you treat a patient with a cholinergic crisis?**

A cholinergic crisis occurs when the patient is overdosed with cholinesterase inhibitors and may show symptoms such as excessive salivation, sweating, abdominal cramps, urinary urgency, bradycardia, muscle fasciculations, or muscle weakness. The treatment is supportive and includes endotracheal intubation, atropine, and cessation of cholinesterase inhibitors until the crisis is over.

5. **What is your plan for postoperative pain? Are there any special considerations?**

Ideally, I would use intrathecal morphine because this can provide prolonged pain control with less respiratory depression than intravenous morphine. If that is not an option, I would use intravenous narcotics sparingly, with NSAIDs and acetaminophen as adjuncts. If an epidural or intercostal nerve block were used, I would avoid ester local anesthetics because they are metabolized by plasma cholinesterase and can worsen symptoms. Instead, I would use amide local anesthetics in reduced doses.

FURTHER READING

Abel M., Eisenkraft J. B. Anesthetic implications of myasthenia gravis. *Mt Sinai J Med* 2002; 69(1–2): 31–37.

Blichfeldt-Lauridsen, L., Hansen, B. D. Anesthesia and myasthenia gravis. *Acta Anaesthesiol Scand* 2012; 56: 17–22.

Miller R. D., Eriksson L. I., Fleisher L. A., Wiener-Kronish J. P. (eds.). *Miller's Anesthesia*, 7th edn. Philadelphia, PA: Churchill Livingstone, 2009.

3

Laryngeal papillomatosis

Aimee Gretchen Kakascik

STEM 1

A 12 year old, 55 kg male from Nigeria is to have surgical excision and ablation of laryngeal papillomas.

HPI: The patient had the diagnosis since early childhood as the human papilloma virus was transmitted to the child during pregnancy. He has had surgical treatments every 6 to 9 weeks since he was 2 years old. He presents today as usual with a soft, hoarse voice and stridor. He is able to go to school, but is unable to participate in any sports or physical education classes.

PMH: His medical history is otherwise negative except that he is positive for human immunodeficiency virus (HIV).

Meds: He takes cidofovir and interferon.

PE: Vital signs – BP 130/78 mmHg, P 105 bpm, RR 22, room air saturation 97%.

General – he is anxious about the procedure.

Airway – Mallampati class II, no loose teeth.

CV – RRR.

Lungs – CTA bilaterally.

Labs: Hct 31%, platelets 50k, Na 135 mEq/L, K 4.1 mEq/L.

Rapid Review Anesthesiology Oral Boards, ed. Ruchir Gupta and Minh Chau Joseph Tran. Published by Cambridge University Press. © Cambridge University Press 2013.

Preoperative

Respiratory

1. **Do you need any additional studies to evaluate the patient's airway?**
   In reviewing his last anesthetic record and confirming with the otolaryngologist that his condition is not worse than before, I would also be interested in any imaging studies such as a neck CT which can help me determine the size, shape, and location of the lesion.

2. **Would you want pulmonary function tests?**
   No. Based on the history given, it appears that the patient has had obstruction at the larynx for years. Thus, a thorough H&P would provide the best information for the management of this child.

3. **What would a flow volume loop of this child look like?**
   The flow volume loop would show flattening of the inspiratory limb, suggesting variable extrathoracic upper airway obstruction or flattening of both the inspiratory and expiratory limbs if the upper airway obstruction is fixed.

Cardiac

4. **Do you have any cardiovascular concerns with this patient? If so, how would you address them?**
   Yes. My concern is that given his long-standing chronic airway obstruction, there is a potential for development of right ventricular hypertrophy and cor pulmonale. I would want a baseline EKG and cardiac echo to determine the presence and extent of any cardiac remodeling that may have occurred in response to the chronic airway obstruction.

5. **What would the EKG of a patient with cor pulmonale show?**
   Right atrial hypertrophy would be seen by peaked P waves in leads II, III, and aVF. Right ventricular hypertrophy would be seen by right axis deviation and a partial or complete right bundle branch block.

Premedication

6. **Would you give any preoperative medication for anxiolysis?**
   Yes, I would give PO midazolam with supplemental oxygen while the child is on telemetry if a preoperative reassuring visit was not enough.

7. **Would you start a peripheral intravenous line before or after induction?**
   If the patient is comfortable with placing an IV line, I would place it before induction. If the patient is fearful of needles I would place it after induction to decrease agitation and the increased oxygen demand with airway obstruction.

Intraoperative

Induction

1. **How will you induce the patient?**
   If the child does not have an IV in place, I will perform a slow inhalational induction with sevoflurane and 100% oxygen while maintaining spontaneous respirations. If there is an IV in place, I will induce with lidocaine, glycopyrrolate, midazolam, and ketamine. In either case, I will have emergency airway equipment in the room and ENT on standby for an emergency tracheostomy if the airway is lost.

2. **The surgeon plans to use carbon dioxide laser to ablate the papillomas. Will you intubate the patient? What are some potential problems with intubation for this case?**
   I would not intubate unless needed as spontaneous ventilation without intubation allows the surgeon to work without interruption and it is preferred to laser-safe endotracheal tubes. Some of the problems with intubation include airway bleeding, airway fire, obstruction of the surgical field, seeding of the papillomas into the distal airways, failure to pass the ETT as a result of the airway obstruction, increased airway resistance (by using a smaller diameter ETT), and further airway scarring from repeated airway manipulations and surgeries.

3. **Do you need any special safety precautions while using a carbon dioxide laser?**
   Flammable surgical drapes should be minimized and wet towels should cover the face, neck, and shoulders to absorb laser energy. The eyes of the patient should be protected with shields or moist gauze pads. Safety glasses should be worn by operating room personnel. To prevent combustion the FiO_2 should be as low as possible and nitrous oxide must not be used. In addition, laser-safe endotracheal tubes should be used with a saline-filled cuff, a fire extinguisher should be present in the room, and a smoke evacuator for the laser and special masks worn by personnel to prevent the spread of virus upon vaporization.

4. **How will you maintain anesthesia, TIVA, or inhalational agents?**
   Given that the patient is not intubated and maintenance of anesthesia with inhalational agents would lead to OR volatile gas contamination and variable depths of anesthesia for the patient during the procedure, I would perform a TIVA technique using propofol infusion (200–300 mcg/kg per min), remifentanil infusion (0.1–0.25 mcg/kg per min), and aerosolized lidocaine.

5. **During the procedure the patient's saturation decreases from 98% to 75%. How will you treat?**
   I would mask ventilate the child with 100% oxygen and if needed have the surgeon intubate the patient until the saturation improves.

6. **The surgeon tells you that the vocal cords are closed. What will you do?**
   I will provide gentle positive mask ventilation with 100% oxygen, and ask the surgeon to apply more aerosolized lidocaine onto the vocal cords after a bolus of propofol is given to deepen the anesthetic. If this does not break the laryngospasm, I would give succinylcholine.

7. **The surgeon has placed an endotracheal tube. While you are ventilating the patient, smoke is seen arising from the airway. What do you do?**
   I am concerned that the endotracheal tube has ignited. I will call for help, stop the flow of oxygen, disconnect the ETT from the gas source, and immediately extubate ensuring that the entire ETT has been removed. A chest radiograph and a bronchoscopy should be performed to determine the extent of injury.

Postoperative

Postoperative treatment of airway fire

1. **The patient was stabilized after the airway fire and mild edema was seen on bronchoscopy. How will you manage the patient?**
   After resecuring the airway with a smaller sized ETT, I will continue with conservative measures by monitoring and giving humidified oxygen, steroids, and racemic epinephrine.

2. **The damage was mild and you decide to take the patient awake to the recovery room. The recovery room nurse calls to tell you that the patient is desaturating with decreased breath sounds bilaterally. Pulse is 140 bpm and blood pressure is 70/40 mmHg. What is your differential diagnosis?**
   My differential diagnosis includes tracheal tear, pneumothorax, airway obstruction, and bronchospasm.

3. **What will you do?**
   I will manually ventilate the patient with 100% oxygen to assess compliance, auscultate for bilateral breath sounds, suction out the ETT, check the circuit for no kinks or occlusions, obtain a CXR, and send an ABG. In the event that my investigation leads me to a surgical etiology (tracheal tear) I will notify the surgeon.

Postoperative carbon dioxide laser complications

4. **A chest radiograph shows bilateral pneumothoraces and subcutaneous emphysema. What is your most likely diagnosis? How do you respond?**
   This is most likely a tracheal tear. I will call for help and prepare to emergently go into the operating room. I will have the surgeon place chest tubes or I would needle decompress the pneumothoraces depending on patient stability. Next, I will have the otolaryngologist replace an endotracheal tube with bronchoscope guidance and prepare for a tracheal repair.

FURTHER READING

Gregory G. A., Andropoulos D. B. (eds.). *Gregory's Pediatric Anesthesia*, 5th edn. Hoboken, NJ: Wiley-Blackwell, 2012.

Kadish H. Thoracic trauma. In: Fleisher G. R., Ludwig S., Henretig F. M. (eds.), *Textbook of Pediatric Emergency Medicine*, 5th edn. Philadelphia, PA: Lippincott, Williams & Wilkins, 2006: 1433.

Hines R. L., Marschall K. E. (eds.). *Stoelting's Anesthesia and Co-Existing Disease*, 5th edn. Philadelphia, PA: Churchill Livingstone, 2008.

4

Sickle cell disease

Ruchir Gupta

STEM 2

A 24 year old female presents for an emergent laparoscopic appendectomy. She has a history of sickle cell disease for which she has received multiple exchange transfusions for vaso-occlusive crises.

Labs: Hb 7 g/dL, WBC 14k/mcL, HbA 30%. Vitals: BP 90/60 mmHg, HR 110 bpm, RR 22, RA SaO_2 98%. She has a 22 g IV with LR hanging.

Preoperative

Transfusion goals

1. **Would you preemptively transfuse this patient?**
   In this particular patient I would transfuse because anemia can precipitate a crisis in a patient with SCD. Additionally this patient is hypotensive and tachycardic, which strongly suggests her anemia is causing instability.

2. **What is your target Hb in this patient?**
   10 g/dL is the recommended Hb in a patient with SCD.

3. **What significance does the HbAA fraction have for you, if any?**
   Ideally, a fraction of at least 50% is desired to prevent sickling in a patient with SCD.

Rapid Review Anesthesiology Oral Boards, ed. Ruchir Gupta and Minh Chau Joseph Tran. Published by Cambridge University Press. © Cambridge University Press 2013.

Crisis

4. **What factors can precipitate a sickle cell crisis?**
Sickle cell crisis can be precipitated by hypo- or hyperthermia, infection, hypotension, stasis, anemia, acidosis, and hypoxia.

5. **What is the pathophysiology of SCD?**
It's caused by a valine to glutamine amino acid substitution which causes a defect in the beta globulin chain.

6. **What are the different types of crises that can occur in a sickle cell patient?**
   (1) Vaso-occlusive due to microinfarcts.
   (2) Aplastic.
   (3) Splenic sequestration.
   (4) Hemolytic (if the patient also has G6P deficiency).
   (5) Acute chest syndrome (respiratory symptoms, fever, pain, hypoxia, infiltrates on CXR).

7. **How would you prevent an SC crisis in this patient?**
I would warm up the OR, rehydrate the patient, transfuse to an Hb of at least 10 g/dL, avoid the use of tourniquets, and prevent hypoxia, hypotension, acidosis, and infection.

Intraoperative

OR setup

1. **How would you prepare the OR for this case?**
I would warm up the OR, use a fluid warmer and Bair Hugger, have blood products available, and place invasive monitors such as a central line and an a-line.

Anesthesia

2. **What monitors would you use?**
In addition to the standard ASA monitors, I would have an a-line to monitor the BP, serial Hct (to avoid anemia), and pH on blood gas (to avoid acidosis). I would also have a central line to better assess volume status, transfusion of blood products, and to keep the patient euvolemic. Lastly, I would want a Foley catheter.

3. **Do you need to have blood products in the OR prior to induction?**
No. Assuming that the patient had already been transfused to a hemoglobin level of 10 g/dL, I can have blood products on standby given that this is a laparoscopic case involving minimal blood loss.

4. **Would you perform a general or regional technique in this patient?**
   I would perform a general anesthetic because this is a laparoscopic procedure on a patient who is a "full stomach" and I would want to secure the airway and have control of her respirations.

Hypotension

5. **As soon as the surgeon insufflates the abdomen, the patient's BP plummets to 60/40 mmHg. What would you do?**
   I would immediately look at my monitor and ensure that the patient is oxygenating and ventilating well and is in sinus rhythm. Assuming she is, I would look at the insufflation pressure and CVP trends. If the CVP number is low it would suggest that she remains intravascularly volume depleted. I would correlate this finding with oscillations in her pulse oximeter tracing with mechanical ventilation and diminished area under the curve of the a-line. Assuming the insufflation pressure is correct, I would temporize her blood pressure with a fluid challenge and neosynephrine. I would also adjust the inspiration:expiration ratio and change to a pressure-controlled ventilation mode. If those maneuvers fail to restore her blood pressure, I would have the surgeon temporarily deflate the abdomen.

Postoperative

Postoperative pain

1. **You are paged to the PACU because the patient is complaining of pain. Why is pain more concerning in this patient than in other patients?**
   Pain is more concerning in this patient since it can signal the onset of an SC crisis.

2. **What will you do?**
   I would immediately go to the bedside and make sure the patient is not hypoxic, hypotensive, or acidotic. Then, I will perform a focused history and physical. From the history, I want to know the pain's location, intensity, and whether it is radiating. I will also look at my anesthesia chart and the nurse's notes to see what pain medicines have been given and if maximum doses of those medicines have been achieved. From the physical, I will inspect the surgical site and make sure there is no abnormal bleeding or drainage at the site. Opioids carry the risk of respiratory depression with resultant respiratory acidosis and hypoxia, both of which can precipitate a crisis. Thus, I will begin pain therapy with non-opioid analgesics such as NSAIDs and Tylenol and gradually move to combination medicines such as Percocet and Vicodin. Finally, after using those, I will begin slow titration of short-acting opioids such as fentanyl.

Acute chest syndrome

3. **On POD #2 the patient develops a productive cough and a low grade fever. There is a left lobe infiltrate on chest X-ray. What is your differential diagnosis?**

Based on this patient's history of sickle cell disease my primary diagnosis would be acute chest syndrome. Other possibilities are pneumonia, ARDS, and pulmonary embolism.

4. **Assuming this was acute chest syndrome, what will be your management?**

Initial treatment begins with supportive measures such as mechanical ventilation, serial ABGs, chest X-rays, and broad spectrum antibiotics. Depending on the clinical course, a simple transfusion or an exchange transfusion may be needed to maintain a hematocrit of 30%.

5. **What precipitates acute chest syndrome?**

The acute chest syndrome is commonly precipitated by noninfectious etiologies such as fat embolism, fluid overload, hypoventilation, in situ thrombosis, bone infarction, and infectious etiologies such as community acquired pneumonia.

FURTHER READING

Gladwin M. T., Schechter A. N., Shelhamer J. H., Ognibene F. P. The acute chest syndrome in sickle cell disease. *Am J Respir Crit Care Med* 1999; 159: 1368–1376.

Platt O. S., Brambilla D. J., Rosse W. F., Milner P. F., Castro O., Steinberg M. H., Klug P. P. Mortality in sickle cell disease: life expectancy and risk factors for early death. *N Engl J Med* 1994; 330: 1639–1644.

5

Liver transplant

Federico Osorio

STEM 1

A 57 year old, 72 kg male is scheduled for a liver transplant.

HPI: The patient suffers from chronic hepatic cirrhosis.

PMH: HTN, hypercholesterolemia.

Meds: He is currently on spironolactone, propranolol, metronidazole, and lactulose.

PE: Vital signs – BP 126/80 mmHg, pulse 104 bpm, RR 28, O_2 92% on RA. Mallampati score is II with a full range of motion. Dentition is normal. Auscultation reveals a systolic murmur due to a systolic anterior motion of the mitral valve (SAM). Fluid-filled abdomen on exam. The rest of the exam is unremarkable.

Labs: Hb 11.3 g/dL, WBC 11k, Na 132 mEq/L, K 4.0 mEq/L.

Preoperative

Cardiac

1. **How would you evaluate this patient's cardiac status?**
   First, a complete medical history and physical examination should be performed. From the history, I would want to know if he has had any episodes of chest pain, shortness of breath, or light-headedness. I would also inquire about his baseline exercise tolerance by determining how many stairs he can climb comfortably. From the physical, I would listen to the heart sounds and

Rapid Review Anesthesiology Oral Boards, ed. Ruchir Gupta and Minh Chau Joseph Tran. Published by Cambridge University Press. © Cambridge University Press 2013.

assess for signs of congestive heart failure such as JVD, pedal edema, pulmonary edema while keeping in mind that fluid overload can also be seen in cirrhosis. Finally, I would look at studies, specifically an EKG, and an echocardiogram because these patients are at high risk for pulmonary hypertension. If available, I would want to know the results of a stress test.

Liver function status

2. **How does this patient's history of cirrhosis affect your anesthetic management?**
   I would ensure the patient has large bore PIV access, a preinduction arterial line, and a central line to allow adequate fluid resuscitation. In terms of induction, this patient most likely has ascites and so must be considered to have a full stomach. Since he could be volume depleted, it would be prudent to use cardiac stable agents for the induction. Higher than normal MAC values may be needed for maintenance because patients with cirrhosis often have a history of alcoholism. Finally, I would also avoid drugs that undergo significant hepatic metabolism.

3. **What are the factors associated with liver disease that lead to the accumulation of ascites?**
   The factors that lead to ascites are hypoalbuminemia, portal hypertension, and water retention (secondary to secretion of antinatriuretic factors and ADH).

4. **What is hepatorenal syndrome?**
   Hepatorenal syndrome is an often fatal condition that is associated with rapid functional renal failure secondary to fulminant liver disease and cirrhosis.

5. **Your resident informs you that there is no recent echocardiogram on file. Would you delay the case?**
   Yes, I would delay because I want to fully understand the severity and symptomatology associated with the systolic murmur because this would affect my anesthetic management. I also want to know if this patient has pulmonary hypertension because severe pulmonary HTN (>50 mmHg) is a contraindication to a transplant.

Intraoperative

Monitors

1. **What kind of monitoring devices are you going to use in this patient?**
   In addition to the standard ASA monitors (pulse oximeter, NIBP, EKG, EtCO$_2$, and temperature) I would place an arterial line, central line catheter (Large 12 Fr.), and a TEE.

2. **Do you have any concerns about the use of TEE in this particular patient?**
   Yes. The use of TEE may cause rupture and bleeding of esophageal varices. However, if extreme caution is exercised during the insertion and manipulation of the TEE probe, the likelihood of this complication has been found to be very low. In this case with the history of SAM and the high hemodynamic variations expected on a liver transplant procedure, I consider that the use of TEE is essential.

Hematologic considerations

3. **Assuming the patient is medically optimized, would you perform an intrathecal morphine injection for perioperative pain control in this patient?**
   No. Liver dysfunction is associated with multiple coagulation derangements (prolonged PT, INR, thrombocytopenia, platelet dysfunction). Regional anesthesia is an unacceptably high-risk procedure for this patient.

4. **Which blood products, if any, would you want in the room?**
   Because these procedures are associated with massive blood loss and coagulopathy, I would want at least 10 units of PRBC, 5–10 units of FFP, 100 units of platelets, and 10 units of cryoprecipitate.

Induction

5. **How would you induce this patient?**
   Because this patient likely has increased intra-abdominal pressure from ascites, I would treat him like a full stomach. Thus, I would premedicate with sodium citrate, metoclopramide, and an H2 antagonist. Then, I would place the patient in reverse Trendelenburg to reduce the risk of any passive regurgitation. Assuming a normal airway, I would perform an RSI with cricoid pressure using etomidate, and succinylcholine after adequate prehydration and placement of a preinduction arterial line.

6. **Immediately after induction, the BP rapidly decreases to 75/40 mmHg, and HR is 80 bpm. What are you going to do?**
   I would immediately place the patient on 100% oxygen, look at the monitors to rule out a malignant arrhythmia, and the pulse oximeter to rule out hypoxia and hypercarbia while feeling for a carotid pulse. Assuming all of these parameters were normal, I would open the fluids and administer a low dose of phenylephrine to improve the BP.

Preanhepatic phase

7. **What are the stages of a liver transplant surgery?**
   (1) Preanhepatic phase: period when the native liver is mobilized and dissected.

(2) Anhepatic phase: period when the native liver is removed.

(3) Reperfusion phase: period during which the new donor liver is anastomosed.

8. **Shortly after the surgeon has made the incision, you notice a very active suctioning sound. The patient starts turning gradually hypotensive although no significant blood loss has occurred. How would you assess? Differential diagnosis? Manage?**

I would immediately look at my vitals and ensure the patient is not hypoxic, hypo- or hypercarbic, or in a malignant rhythm. Assuming all of this was normal, the most common initial cause of hypotension at the early stages of liver transplant is hypovolemia due to the combination of the vasodilatory effects of the induction agents and the drainage of ascites. Thus, I would administer a bolus of a colloid-containing solution, and continue giving boluses according to the CVP values and the appearance of the heart cavities on the TEE.

Anhepatic stage

9. **Twenty-five minutes into the anhepatic phase you notice a sustained period of hypotension, with no significant increases in blood loss. CVP = 11 mmHg, H/H = 10 g/dL/L, 30%. How would you evaluate this situation?**

First, I would look at the patient's other vitals to make sure they are stable. During the anhepatic stage blood loss is not the typical cause of hypotension, especially after having a normal CVP value. After ruling out a mechanical cause of the problem by looking over the surgical field and asking the surgical team to check for sponges and evaluating suction containers, I would focus on contractility issues. First, I would review the electrocardiogram trace looking for prolongation of the QT interval (hypocalcemia) and ST interval (changes during acute ischemic events). I'll also look at my TEE to evaluate for regional wall motion abnormalities +/− global hypokinesia.

10. **What is the difference between the "traditional technique" and the "piggyback" technique during the anhepatic phase? How do they affect your anesthetic management?**

In the traditional technique, the surgeon performs a complete vascular occlusion by clamping the IVC, suprahepatic vena cava, hepatic artery, and the portal vein. As a result, venous return decreases by 50–60% and severe hypotension with a compensatory tachycardia may occur from the low CO. To prevent this, venovenous bypass (VVBP) would have to be initiated and the complications associated with VVBP such as arm edema, air embolism, and vascular injury would have to be treated. The alternative is for me to volume load the patient with a target CVP of 10–20 mmHg and administer vasopressor boluses prior to clamping of the vessels. In the piggyback technique, the vena cava is partially occluded, making the surgery more challenging but eliminating the need for VVBP or the hemodynamic fluctuations encountered with the traditional technique.

Reperfusion stage

11. **The surgeon notifies you that he/she is about to "reperfuse." How would you prepare for this?**

    Reperfusing the transplanted liver is one of the most critical moments of the operation, because the recipient's blood will flush through the new liver and force multiple metabolic products into the main circulation. This will lead to a decrease in cardiac contractility, CO, SVR, and abrupt rises in pulmonary vascular resistance and serum hydrogen and potassium ion concentrations.

    I would prepare by keeping the patient's intravascular volume optimized, checking the ABG and H/H to correct any acid–base electrolyte disorder, and transfuse according to hemodynamic and H/H levels. I would have pressors, calcium, insulin, sodium bicarbonate, and blood products in line ready for use. Once the patient's status is optimized, I would notify the surgeon to start the reperfusion process.

12. **What is meant by the "reperfusion syndrome?"**

    Reperfusion syndrome is hemodynamic instability of unknown mechanism usually occurring during the first 5 minutes of reperfusion that is associated with hyperkalemia and hemodynamic fluctuations such as hypotension, bradycardia, elevated PAP, and supraventricular tachycardia.

Postoperative

Postoperative bleeding

1. **You are paged to the SICU because the nurse had just noticed that the drains from the abdominal cavity have been filling up rapidly. What should you do at this point?**

    I would immediately go to the patient's bedside and evaluate his vital signs to make sure they are stable while asking the nurse to notify the surgeon. I would send an ABG, H/H, and TEG samples. If hypotension was present I would give a bolus of 500 mL of LR immediately, as well as a dose of phenylephrine to recover the BP.

Coagulopathy and anemia

2. **While you are administering the first bolus of fluids, the laboratory calls to inform you that the TEG maximum amplitude value is below the normal values. Hb = 9.2 g/dL, pH = 7.32, $PaCO_2$ = 53 mmHg, BE = −2. CVP = 4 cmH_2O, BP = 98/54 mmHg. What would you do?**

The low MA value suggests to me an issue related to the platelet component. Thus I would start transfusing two bags of platelets, watching closely the CVP value since a high CVP may lead to congestion of the new liver and trigger further bleeding and/or graft dysfunction. The other results suggest anemia, which can be worsened by the transfusion of non-red blood cells containing fluids. Therefore, I would prepare the patient for blood transfusion, making sure of the availability of 5 units of blood. The ABG suggests the presence of mild respiratory acidosis, so I would adjust the mechanical ventilation by increasing the respiratory rate or tidal volume as tolerated.

3. **After the transfusion of 2 units of platelets, the patient's nurse calls you to tell you the patient's bleeding had initially improved but is now worsening again. How do you respond?**
   I would immediately evaluate the patient at the bedside. I will check vital signs to verify stability. Based on the clinical presentation of recurring hemorrhage and the findings from the TEG results, the diagnosis of fibrinolysis is more clear. At this point, I would order a dose of intravenous aminocaproic acid and check the level of fibrinogen to determine if a transfusion of cryoprecipitate is required.

FURTHER READING

Hines R. L., Marschall K. E. (eds.) *Stoelting's Anesthesia and Co-Existing Disease*, 5th edn. Philadelphia, PA: Saunders Elsevier, 2008.

O'Riordan J., O'Beirne H. A, Young Y., Bellamy M. C. Effects of desflurane and isoflurane on splanchnic microcirculation during major surgery. *Br J Anaesth* 1997; 78(1): 95–96.

Prasad S., Dhiman R. K., Duseja A., Chawla Y. K., Sharma A., Agarwal R. Lactulose improves cognitive functions and health-related quality of life in patients with cirrhosis who have minimal hepatic encephalopathy. *Hepatology* 2007; 45(3): 549–559.

Randolph H., Steadman, M. D. Anesthesia for liver transplant surgery. *Anesthesiol Clin North Am* 2004; 22: 687–711.

6

Renal transplantation

Ruchir Gupta, Sheryl Glassman, and Anita Gupta

STEM 2

A 55 year old female is scheduled for a cadaveric kidney transplant harvested 16 hours ago. She underwent dialysis 25 hours ago. She has a history of diabetes mellitus, hypertension, and coronary artery disease. Medications include: glipizide, metoprolol, and alprazolam. VS: HR 75, BP 180/90 mmHg, RR 24, RA saturation 97%.

Labs: Hb 11.3 g/dL, Plt 235k, WBC 10.1k/mcL, Na 140 mEq/L, K 5.2 mEq/L.

Preoperative

End-stage renal disease

1. **What are the systemic manifestations of chronic renal failure?**
   Chronic renal failure (CRF) has effects on multiple organ systems:
   Cardiac: patients are at risk for HTN, CHF, cardiomyopathy, CAD, and hyperdynamic circulation.
   Pulmonary: patients may have pulmonary edema.
   GI: gastroparesis, gastritis, and pancreatitis.
   Hematologic: anemia, coagulopathy, metabolic acidosis, hyperkalemia, hyperphosphatemia, hypocalcemia, and hyperuricemia.
   Neurologic: encephalopathy, peripheral neuropathy, seizures, myoclonus, and asterixis.

2. **What hematologic issues are you concerned about in this patient?**
   In addition to a baseline chronic anemia, I am concerned that this patient may have a coagulopathy because many patients with CRF have thrombocytopathia and decreased prothrombin levels.

Rapid Review Anesthesiology Oral Boards, ed. Ruchir Gupta and Minh Chau Joseph Tran. Published by Cambridge University Press. © Cambridge University Press 2013.

3. **Will you order any additional preoperative tests in this patient?**
   Yes. I would want an EKG, chest radiograph, coagulation profile, liver function enzymes, bilirubin, albumin.

Hyperkalemia

4. **Will you delay the case to correct this patient's serum potassium level?**
   No. Chronic hyperkalemia secondary to the renal failure is an expected finding with this patient. As long as she was not symptomatic, I would not delay the case. I would have medications such as calcium, insulin, glucose, bicarbonate, and beta-agonist in the OR prior to induction, however.

5. **What if the patient's repeat serum potassium comes back at 6.0 mEq/L? Will you delay the case then?**
   Yes. At 6.0 mEq/L the serum K⁺ is at a life-threatening level and can lead to ventricular fibrillation and asystole. I would delay the case and immediately begin treatment with calcium, insulin, bicarbonate, beta-agonists, and glucose.

6. **The surgeon says that a serum K⁺ of 6.0 mEq/L is a normal laboratory finding in a patient with renal failure and this is an emergency procedure. How will you respond?**
   I will inform the surgeon of two things:
   (1) Renal transplants are not emergent cases. Cadaveric kidneys can be maintained for 36–48 hours to optimize the patient and preoperative optimization will ensure a better outcome for the patient.
   (2) While some patients with ESRD do suffer from chronic hyperkalemia, a value of 6.0 mEq/L can be lethal and thus cannot be considered a normal finding. At this level, the patient may develop a malignant cardiac rhythm at any time.

Medications

7. **The patient informs you that she did not take any of her medications this morning. How would you manage this patient's home medication regimen prior to bringing her to the operating room?**
   This patient is currently on glipizide for DM, metoprolol for HTN, and alprazolam for presumed anxiety. I would hold her glipizide because oral hypoglycemics should not be administered since the patient will be NPO and hypoglycemia may result from its administration. Conversely, I would continue her metoprolol because any patient on long-term beta blocker therapy should continue it to reduce the risk of morbidity and mortality during such procedures. Finally, in terms of alprazolam, I would ask the patient to take her normal dose so that she doesn't have any symptoms of withdrawal or anxiety prior to arriving to the OR. Additionally, if she does appear anxious, I could titrate in a low dose of midazolam prior to bringing her to the OR.

Premedication

8. **Would you administer any premedications to this patient?**

It depends. If this patient appeared anxious, I would begin with verbal reassurance. If she continued to be anxious, I would consider administering a low dose of midazolam. Next, because this patient is at risk for gastroparesis, I would administer sodium citrate as well as promotility agents such as metoclopramide, which will promote gastric emptying.

Intraoperative

Regional vs. general anesthesia techniques

1. **Could you do this case under regional?**

No. This patient likely has a coagulopathy secondary to uricemia leading to decreased vWF levels. Thus, I will want to avoid neuraxial techniques completely.

Monitors

2. **How would you monitor this patient?**

I would place the standard ASA monitors, a neuromuscular blockade monitor, preinduction arterial line and a central line to optimize intravascular volume and follow CVP trends.

Induction

3. **How would you induce this patient?**

Assuming the patient has a reassuring airway, I would preoxygenate with 100% O_2 and do a rapid sequence induction with fentanyl, etomidate, and succinylcholine. I would perform a rapid sequence induction technique to reduce the risk of aspiration in this patient, likely to have gastroparesis secondary to chronic renal insufficiency.

Maintenance

4. **Assuming you decided to do this case under general anesthesia, what agents would you use for maintenance?**

I would use a balanced anesthetic technique with a volatile anesthetic, an opioid, and a muscle relaxant. In terms of my inhalation agent, I would use desflurane because it does not have nephrotoxic potential and has rapid wash-in and wash-out time. I would avoid sevoflurane because its metabolism can produce nephrotoxic agents such as compound A and fluoride. Opioids can be used to maintain analgesia. In terms of opioids, I would avoid morphine and meperidine because both depend on renal clearance and have active metabolites that can accumulate (morphine-3-glucuronide and morphine-6-glucuronide and normeperidine respectively). Morphine-6-glucuronide accumulation can lead to worsening of respiratory depression. Normeperidine accumulation can lead to neurotoxic effects such as seizure activity. Finally, for neuromuscular blockade I would use cisatracurium since metabolism and elimination are independent of the renal pathway.

Preparation for graft attachment

5. **The surgeon informs you that he is about to clamp the iliac vessels. What medications would you administer at this time?**
   I would administer heparin prior to clamping (to prevent clotting), and have the surgeon inject verapamil or papaverine into the graft arteries prior to revascularization (to prevent arterial vasospasm) and mannitol/furosemide after graft reperfusion (to induce diuresis).

Renal graft reperfusion

6. **The kidney graft vessels and ureter are anastomosed and the clamp is now removed. The patient's blood pressure quickly plummets to 77/38 mmHg. How do you respond?**
   I would immediately check the patient's other vital signs including heart rate, pulse, end-tidal CO_2, oxygen saturation, and EKG for any malignant arrhythmia. Hypotension immediately following unclamping is most likely due to the wash-out of vasoactive substances from the renal graft. Treatment would be primarily supportive. Thus, assuming all of my other vital signs were stable, I would open my fluids wide, administer pressors such as phenylephrine or ephedrine, and send an ABG with electrolytes.

7. **The EKG monitor shows peaked T waves. What is your response?**
   This is most likely due to hyperkalemia from the preservative fluid of the new kidney. Thus, I would administer calcium gluconate for myocardial protection and then administer insulin, glucose, bicarbonate, and a beta-agonist to decrease the serum levels of K^+.

Postoperative

Extubation

1. **Will you extubate this patient?**
   It depends on the clinical course. If the patient demonstrated hemodynamic stability with stable vital signs, was awake and alert, followed commands,

was pulling in adequate tidal volumes (>6 mL/kg), was fully reversed, and the operation was devoid of large fluid shifts, I would extubate. However, if the patient developed some unforeseen intraoperative event or/and massive fluid shifts and was not able to breathe on her own, I would prefer to leave the patient intubated overnight.

Postoperative oliguria

2. **You are paged STAT to the PACU for decreased urine output. What is your differential?**
Oliguria can be categorized as prerenal, intrarenal, and postrenal. Prerenal is due to hypoperfusion which is usually caused by hypovolemia. Thus, I will check my inputs/outputs to assess how much fluid the patient has been given, my CVP readings if I have a central line, and send for electrolytes to assess for signs of dehydration such as hypernatremia. I will also look at my skin turgor and the mucous membranes. Postrenal pathology is usually due to a kinked Foley catheter or bladder obstruction. Intrarenal is often due to the presence of nephrotoxic substances. A UA with casts would be helpful in confirming the diagnosis. Additionally, this patient may be experiencing graft rejection, toxic injury, or vessel occlusion.

3. **What are some laboratory differences between prerenal and renal oliguria?**
Common indices to differentiate prerenal and renal oliguria include urine osmolality, urine sodium, fractional excretion of sodium (FeNA), and urine to serum creatinine ratio. Urine osmolarity (mOsm/L) is greater than 500 in patients with prerenal etiology and less than 400 in patients with renal etiology. Urine sodium is less than 20 mEq/L in prerenal patients and greater than 40 mEq/L in patients with renal etiology. The urine:serum creatinine ratio is greater than 40 in prerenal etiology patients and less than 20 in patients with renal etiology. The BUN:creatinine ratio in prerenal etiology patients is greater than 20 and often less than 10–15 in renal etiology patients. FeNA, measured as a percentage, is less than 1% in prerenal patients and greater than 2% in renal patients.

Nausea

4. **You are paged from the postoperative care unit because the patient is complaining of nausea. How will you respond?**
Nausea is possible from several etiologies. My first response would be to rule out hypoxia, hypoventilation, and hypotension. I would also evaluate for anxiety, postoperative pain, and opioid side effect. Assuming all of this was normal, I would administer a dose of a 5HT3 blocker such as Zofran.

FURTHER READING

Barash P. G., Cullen B. F., Stoelting R. K., Cahalan M., Stock C. M. (eds.). *Clinical Anesthesia*, 6th edn. Philadelphia, PA: Lippincott Williams & Wilkins, 2009.

Miller R. D., Eriksson L. I., Fleisher L. A., Wiener-Kornish J. P., Young W. L. (eds.). *Miller's Anesthesia*, 7th edn. Philadelphia, PA: Churchill Livingstone Elsevier, 2010.

Yao F., Fontes M. L., Malhotra V. (eds.). *Yao and Artusio's Anesthesiology: Problem-Oriented Patient Management*, 7th edn. Philadelphia, PA: Lippincott Williams & Wilkins, 2011.

Thyroidectomy

Ruchir Gupta

STEM 1

A 35 year old female, 55 kg, is scheduled for resection of a goiter. Patient has had dysphagia and dyspnea for the past month.

PMH: Asthma.

Meds: Albuterol, propylthiouracil.

Allergies: NKDA.

PE: VS   HR 130 bpm, BP 180/95 mmHg, RR 20.

> Airway – Mallampati II, full cervical range of motion.

> CV – tachycardic.

> Pulmonary – clear to auscultation.

Labs: Hb 11.2 g/dL, platelets 280k, Na 135 mEq/L.

Preoperative

Hemodynamics

1. **Is this patient ready for surgery?**
   No. This patient is displaying signs of thyrotoxicosis, most likely secondary to increased secretion of the thyroid hormone from the goiter. I would delay the case until this patient is medically managed and made euthyroid.

Rapid Review Anesthesiology Oral Boards, ed. Ruchir Gupta and Minh Chau Joseph Tran. Published by Cambridge University Press. © Cambridge University Press 2013.

2. **The surgeon says this is an emergency case. How will you respond?**

I would inform the surgeon that this is not an emergency case. Thyroidectomy is an elective procedure and this patient needs to be medically managed prior to taking her to the OR to prevent life-threatening hemodynamic changes. Currently, this patient is receiving only propylthiouracil. I would substitute or add methimazole to her regimen for 6–8 weeks because propylthiouracil by itself is not accomplishing the goal. I would also want this patient to take potassium iodide for 10–14 days.

Beta blockers

3. **Are beta blockers helpful in these types of patients? Would you use it in this particular patient?**

Beta blockers do not affect the underlying thyroid pathology but are helpful in reducing the signs and symptoms of thyroid pathology such as hypertension and tachycardia. However, in this particular patient, I would want to only administer B1 selective agents such as metoprolol and avoid drugs that block B2 as these could exacerbate her asthma.

Optimization

4. **If this were a true surgical emergency, what steps would you take to prepare this patient for surgery?**

I would take steps to reduce the possibility of developing a thyroid storm. I would administer antithyroid drugs such as methimazole and propylthiouracil to decrease thyroid hormone synthesis, iopanoic acid to reduce T_3 levels, and glucocorticoids to block peripheral conversion of T_4 to T_3.

Airway

5. **The patient returns 2 months later with HR of 88 bpm, BP 110/70 mmHg, RR 12. How would you examine this patient's airway?**

I would perform a focused history and physical. From the history, I would ask this patient about her dysphagia and dyspnea, assessing whether it has been getting worse or is stable, any exacerbating/alleviating factors, any prior intubations, and if she had had these symptoms at the time. From the physical, I would perform an external airway exam to assess if there is any neck compression by the goiter. I would also perform an internal exam to see if there is any gross deviation in the oropharynx. Most importantly, I will want a flow volume loop to assess if there is any intra/extrathoracic compression and also look at any CT scans that may help me quantify the size and extent of the tumor.

Antithyroid therapy

6. **Would you continue this patient's antithyroid medicines on the morning of surgery or would you ask the patient to discontinue them before?**
   All antithyroid medications should be continued until the morning of surgery.

Intraoperative

Monitoring

1. **Does this patient need a PA catheter for the case?**
   Based on the information given, I do not think this patient needs a PA catheter at this time because I can monitor this patient's hemodynamic status accurately with my standard ASA monitors as well as a central line and a-line if necessary. A PA catheter increases this patient's risk of infection, pneumothorax, vascular/cardiac injury, and bleeding. Thus, in this case I do not believe the benefits outweigh the risks.

2. **Would you place an a-line? Why?**
   Yes. In this patient I would want an a-line which I could use for beat-to-beat monitoring of the blood pressure at critical times during the induced hypotension period, serial ABGs, and H/H assessments.

Airway

3. **How are you going to secure the airway?**
   Given the patient's history of dysphagia and dyspnea and presumed airway mass effect from the goiter, I would perform an awake fiberoptic intubation.

Anesthesia

4. **Your resident suggests using ketamine to keep the patient spontaneously breathing during the FOI. How do you respond?**
   Yes, but only if the patient cannot tolerate an AFOI technique despite adequate airway topicalization with nebulized lidocaine and cetacaine spray and if she remains euthyroid on the day of surgery since ketamine can raise her blood pressure and heart rate.

Bleeding

5. **Does this patient need a higher MAC for anesthetic maintenance?**
   No. MAC values are the same for a euthyroid patient as for a hyperthyroid patient.

6. **Midway through the case, the surgeon informs you that he accidentally cut into an artery and the patient is losing massive amounts of blood. The patient's BP now reads 85/70 mmHg. What will you do?**

   I will immediately place the patient on 100% oxygen and look at my other vital signs and make sure the patient is not hypoxic, hypercarbic, or in a malignant arrhythmia. Next I will open my fluids wide while drawing a STAT ABG to determine an H/H. I will also call for blood and administer a direct acting agent such as phenylephrine as a temporizing measure.

7. **Can you use ephedrine as a temporizing measure?**

   Yes, but only if the patient is made euthyroid. Hyperthyroid patients may have exaggerated response to indirect agents.

Postoperative

Extubation

1. **Will you extubate this patient?**

   It depends. If the case went uneventfully, the patient was fully reversed and following commands, and taking adequate tidal volumes, I would extubate. If, however, this was a complicated case with massive transfusion requirements, swelling at the surgical site, and the patient was not able to take adequate tidal volumes, I would leave the patient intubated and sedated overnight.

Postoperative stridor

2. **You are paged from the PACU because the patient has developed stridor. What is your differential?**

   My differential diagnosis is recurrent laryngeal nerve injury, laryngospasm, tracheomalacia, hematoma formation at the surgical site, inadequate muscle relaxant reversal, and residual anesthetic.

3. **How would you determine if the cause of the injury was bilateral recurrent laryngeal nerve damage?**

   To assess for bilateral RLN injury, I would ask the patient to say "EE." In bilateral injury, the patient would be aphonic.

4. **A STAT electrolyte panel reveals a low serum calcium level. What do you think could have caused this?**

   Inadvertent removal of the parathyroid glands can result in hypocalcemia with resulting respiratory distress. Usually this does not manifest until 24 hours postoperatively.

5. **What is Chvostek's sign?**

   Chvostek's sign is facial nerve excitability due usually to hypocalcemia.

FURTHER READING

Atchabahian A., Gupta R. (eds.). *The Anesthesia Guide*. New York: McGraw-Hill Publishing, 2013.

Hines R. L., Marschall, K. E. (eds.). *Stoelting's Anesthesia and Co-Existing Disease*, 5th edn. Philadelphia, PA: Saunders, 2008.

8

Carcinoid tumor

Xiaodong Bao

STEM 2

A 50 year old, 60 kg female is scheduled for resection of an abdominal carcinoid tumor. She has a medical history of COPD from chronic smoking, hypertension, hyperlipidemia, and decreased activity level. Medications include HCTZ, lisinopril, and simvastatin. She was diagnosed with the carcinoid tumor with hepatic metastasis 3 months ago and has been placed on octreotide. BP 118/77 mmHg, HR 76 bpm, RR 14, O_2 saturation 97% on RA. Labs: Na 138 mEq/L, K 3.2 mEq/L, Hb 12.2 g/dL.

Preoperative

Carcinoid tumor

1. **How would you evaluate this patient's carcinoid?**
   First, I would determine if the tumor is functional or nonfunctional through a focused history and physical. Functional tumors secrete bioactive substances causing a wide range of symptoms including flushing and diarrhea, whereas nonfunctional tumors do not. Thus, from the history, I would ask if the patient has experienced any bronchospasm, diarrhea, dramatic swings in BP, or any increased heart rate or palpitations (SVT). From the physical, I would examine the patient for any evidence of bronchospasm and any heart murmurs since carcinoid tumors can be associated with right heart lesions. Next, I would look at any imaging studies to see where the tumor is located and its overall size.

2. **Do you expect this patient's carcinoid to be functional?**
   Most patients with intestinal carcinoid tumors do not have symptoms because the vasoactive substances are cleared by the portal circulation. However, given

Rapid Review Anesthesiology Oral Boards, ed. Ruchir Gupta and Minh Chau Joseph Tran. Published by Cambridge University Press. © Cambridge University Press 2013.

that this patient has hepatic metastasis, there is a likelihood the tumors are functional.

3. **How is a carcinoid tumor diagnosed?**
Assuming the patient is symptomatic, carcinoid can be confirmed with urinary 5-hydroxyindoleacetic acid and serum levels of chromogranin A.

Cardiac

4. **How would you evaluate the patient's cardiac status preoperatively?**
First, I would start with a detailed history and physical. From the history, I would want to quantify this patient's decreased baseline activity level. Also, any recent episodes of chest pain or shortness of breath would be elicited. From the physical, I would want to know if this patient has heart murmurs or signs of CHF such as edema, or elevated JVD, since these patients are at risk for right-sided valvular lesions and even right-sided heart failure. Finally, I would look at any studies including a baseline EKG, echo, or recent stress test.

5. **What structural changes would you expect to find on a cardiac echo?**
Tricuspid regurgitation is the most frequent phenomenon. Tricuspid stenosis may occur also. Pulmonary insufficiency or stenosis has been reported as well. All these could lead to right-sided heart failure.

Pulmonary

6. **How would you evaluate this patient's pulmonary function?**
First, I would obtain a detailed history and physical. From the history, I would assess frequency/duration of cough, sputum production, dyspnea, exercise tolerance, oxygen requirement, cyanosis, clubbing, and any history of pneumonia. From the physical, I would focus on the patient's breathing pattern, especially any use of accessory muscles. I would also auscultate for wheezing, rhonchi, or rales. Finally, I would look at a baseline CXR and EKG to evaluate for possible cor pulmonale.

7. **Would you obtain PFTs?**
No. PFTs have not been shown to affect anesthetic management in most cases. For this patient, I can obtain most of my information from a detailed H&P.

Metabolic

8. **What substances are released by a carcinoid tumor?**
Carcinoid tumors are derived from enterochromaffin cells that make up the amine precursor uptake and decarboxylation (APUD) system. They may release an array of mediators, including serotonin, histamine, catecholamines, tachykinin, bradykinin, prostaglandin, and vasoactive intestinal peptide. The

substances can cause flushing, diarrhea, abdominal pain, bronchospasm, palpitation, hypertension or hypotension, and heart failure.

9. **What are your anesthetic concerns for a patient with a carcinoid tumor?**
   In addition to the routine cardiac and pulmonary precautions, I am concerned about the precipitation of a carcinoid crisis. Thus, I would ask the patient if there are specific triggers for her carcinoid. Stress, anxiety, exercise, or certain foods high in serotonin such as coffee, cheese, alcohol, bananas are known triggers for carcinoid symptoms. I would be sure to reduce preoperative anxiety, as well as stress from the intubation, surgery, or pain. I would also be cautious about histamine releasing medications and indirect acting agents such as a beta-agonist, which can increase the release of vasoactive substance from the tumor. Finally, I will be vigilant about direct surgical tumor manipulation since that can trigger a carcinoid crisis.

Intraoperative

Monitoring

1. **What kind of monitors are you going to use for this patient?**
   In addition to the standard ASA monitors, I would like to have a preinduction a-line. I would also want a central line to have adequate IV access as well as to volume resuscitate during a carcinoid crisis.

2. **What is the effect of carcinoid tumor on MAC value?**
   Increased serotonin level will result in lower MAC value and delayed awakening. The higher the serotonin level, the lower the MAC value.

Induction

3. **How would you induce this patient?**
   My goal is to maintain hemodynamic stability and reduce the risk of carcinoid crisis by avoiding hypotension, catecholamine secretion, and histamine release. Thus, assuming a normal airway, I would perform a slow controlled induction with fentanyl, etomidate, and rocuronium.

Maintenance

4. **How would you maintain anesthesia for the patient?**
   I would use a balanced technique using oxygen/air, isoflurane, fentanyl, and rocuronium.

Hypotension

5. **After the incision, the patient suddenly becomes hypotensive. What is your differential diagnosis? How would you manage?**

   My differential includes hypovolemia secondary to blood loss, cardiogenic shock from acute arrhythmia, RV failure, anaphylaxis, anesthetic overdose, and a carcinoid crisis. I would quickly look at my VS to make sure the patient is not hypoxic, hypocarbic, or in a malignant arrhythmia. If the patient has been on preoperative octreotide treatment, hypotension is unlikely due to a carcinoid crisis. I would immediately open my IV fluids wide, give phenylephrine or vasopressin as a temporizing measure, and lighten my anesthetic. If I think the hypotension is due to release of vasoactive mediators, I would give an additional 50–100 mcg octreotide every 5–10 min up to 1 mg and hydrocortisone. Aprotinin, a kallikrein inhibitor, has been used to treat hypotension refractory to octreotide as well.

Bronchospasm

6. **In the middle of the case, you notice that the patient's peak airway pressure suddenly rises. What would you do?**

   I would quickly check my vital signs making sure they were all stable. I would then take the patient off the ventilator and begin manual ventilation to assess for airway compliance. I would also check my apparatus to ensure there is no kinking or occlusion of the circuit or ETT as well as ETT migration. I would then increase my anesthetic depth in an effort to break the bronchospasm. If the peak airway pressure does not improve despite these measures and it is associated with skin flushing and manipulation of tumor by the surgeon, I would give an extra 100 mcg of octreotide bolus.

7. **What metabolic disturbance would you expect to see from a patient on an octreotide infusion?**

   Octreotide can cause glucose intolerance.

Postoperative

Pain

1. **How do you plan to manage the patient's pain postoperatively?**

   I would administer a fentanyl PCA for this patient to help with the pain control and to minimize histamine release. In addition, a neuraxial technique such as an epidural can be used with caution since hypotension can also precipitate a crisis.

Octreotide

2. Your medical student asks if you want to discard the octreotide infusion to simplify patient transfer to the ICU now that the patient is stable. Your response?

There is no general agreement on the tapering of the octreotide infusion. The tapering regimen depends on severity of tumor, duration of surgery, type of procedure, the chances of undetected metastases, and residual effects of carcinoid tumor mediators. However, literature recommends tapering octreotide over a week postoperatively.

FURTHER READING

Castillo J. G, Filsoufi F., Adams D. H, Raikhelkar J., Zaku B., Fischer G. W. Management of patients undergoing multivalvular surgery for carcinoid heart disease: the role of the anaesthetist. *Br J Anaesth* 2008; 101(5): 618–626.

Mancuso K., Kaye A. D, Boudreaux J. P, Fox C. J., Lang P., Kalarickal P. L., Gomez S., Primeaux P. J. Carcinoid syndrome and perioperative anesthetic considerations. *J Clin Anesth* 2011; 23: 329–341.

9

Pheochromocytoma

Stanley Yuan and John Cooley

STEM 1

A 74 year old, 56 kg female presents for resection of an abdominal pheochromocytoma. She has had recurrent hypertensive episodes for the past month and has recently begun to experience palpitations and sweating.

PMH: Coronary artery disease.

PSH: Cardiac stents placed 5 years ago.

Allergies: NKDA.

PE: VS – P 88 bpm, RR 14, BP 121/76 mmHg, RA saturation 98%,

Airway – Mallampati II, full cervical range of motion.

CV – regular rate and rhythm.

Pulmonary – clear to auscultation.

Labs: Hb 14.2 g/dL, Plt 240k, K+ 3.3 mEq/L.

Preoperative

Medical clearance

1. **How would you determine if this patient is optimized for surgery?**
   I would first perform a full history and physical. Initial assessment should include volume status, blood pressure trends, and symptoms of shortness of breath and chest discomfort. I would also want to know if she has been taking alpha- followed by beta-antagonist agents. This sequence is crucial

Rapid Review Anesthesiology Oral Boards, ed. Ruchir Gupta and Minh Chau Joseph Tran. Published by Cambridge University Press. © Cambridge University Press 2013.

to avoid hypertensive crisis from unopposed alpha action. According to the Roizen criteria, adequate blockade includes supine blood pressure under 160/90 mmHg, presence of orthostatic hypotension not greater than 80/45 mmHg, electrocardiogram without ST segment or T wave changes, and no more than one PVC every 5 minutes.

2. **How would you evaluate her cardiac status?**
   I would elicit from the patient what her baseline level of functioning is. Specifically, whether she is able to walk up and down a flight of stairs without any discomfort, any recent episodes of chest pain, shortness of breath, or light-headedness. I would also look at a baseline EKG as well as the results of any echocardiogram or stress test that may have been recently done. If time permitted, I would want to talk to her cardiologist as well.

3. **Is there any additional workup you require the patient to have prior to surgery?**
   Currently, this patient has an elevated H/H which is indicative of hypovolemia. I would also want serum electrolytes to assess renal function and glucose level, a chest X-ray to identify cardiomegaly or COPD and a recent EKG to compare it to any old one. Since her CABG was 5 years ago, a recent echocardiogram and stress test are indicated.

Diagnosis

4. **How is pheochromocytoma diagnosed?**
   Pheochromocytomas are endocrine tumors that release catecholamines. With clinical suspicion, plasma metanephrine testing has the highest sensitivity for detecting pheochromocytomas. Elevated urinary VMA can also be used. With positive biochemical markers, computed tomography or magnetic resonance imaging can be performed to localize the tumor with or without iodine-131-labeled meta-iodobenzylguanidine.

5. **What is the rule of 10s in pheochromocytomas?**
   The rule of 10s with pheochromocytomas is that 10% are bilateral, 10% are extra-adrenal, 10% are malignant, and 10% are familial.

Hypotension

6. **The patient suddenly becomes hypotensive and tachycardic preoperatively while changing into her gown. What do you do?**
   I would immediately check the vital signs and make sure the patient is adequately oxygenating and ventilating, and no malignant arrhythmia is developing with a 12-lead EKG. Assuming that was normal, I would rule out myocardial ischemia by asking targeted questions. If the patient is hypovolemic, I would administer 500 mL volume bolus with the patient placed supine on a stretcher. If no

obvious underlying etiology was found, I would regard it as a vasovagal response and treat it accordingly.

Intraoperative

Monitor

1. **How would you monitor this patient?**

   I would place the patient on standard ASA monitors with a five-lead electrocardiogram. A preinduction intra-arterial catheter is indicated to avoid blood pressure swings. With the nature of this surgery and fluid shift, central venous access is also important for both central venous pressure monitoring and the administration of blood products and medications. I would also place a pulmonary arterial catheter or a transesophageal echocardiogram depending on her preoperative cardiac workup.

Induction

2. **How would you induce this patient?**

   Assuming a normal airway, I would preoxygenate this patient with 100% oxygen, and perform a slow controlled induction with fentanyl and etomidate, and once I saw I could mask ventilate, I would administer rocuronium. I would be looking at my arterial line reading during the induction, and have pressors and dilators on standby to treat abrupt changes in blood pressure.

3. **During direct laryngoscopy, you are unable to visualize the vocal cords. What are you going to do?**

   I would mask ventilate with 100% oxygen and call for help. Assuming I am able to ventilate the patient, I would attempt direct laryngoscopy once again after repositioning the airway and switching blades. If I couldn't mask ventilate, I would place an LMA and attempt to ventilate the patient via the LMA.

4. **Are there other options besides general anesthesia for this surgery?**

   There are documented case reports of successful regional technique for open pheochromocytoma resection. One should focus on an anesthetic plan that is most comfortable and familiar. Communication with the surgical team is imperative. If this is an open anterior transabdominal approach, an epidural catheter can be inserted at around T8 level for both intraoperative and postoperative analgesia.

5. **What medications, if any, would you avoid during this case?**

   I would avoid drugs that
   (1) would stimulate the tumor cells – succinylcholine by causing fasciculations, histamine-releasing drugs such as morphine and atracurium;

(2) can cause an increase in sympathetic activity – such as atropine, ketamine, and ephedrine.

Hypertension

6. **Forty-five minutes into the case, during tumor manipulation the BP increases to 210/105 mmHg. How will you respond?**
   I would immediately look at my other vital signs and rule out hypoxia, hypercarbia, or a malignant rhythm while asking the surgeon to stop tumor manipulation. Highest on my differential is hypertension due to release of catecholamines from tumor manipulation. Thus, assuming my other vital signs are normal, I would immediately begin an infusion of sodium nitroprusside. Other agents that can also be utilized are nitroglycerin and nicardipine, and if tachyarrhythmias are present, I would give esmolol.

Hypotension

7. **Patient is hypotensive immediately after the tumor is resected. What do you do?**
   Hypotension is common after tumor resection. I would first confirm the tracing on the intra-arterial line and ensure her other vital signs are stable. If the arterial line reading is true and other vital signs are stable, all vasodilators should be discontinued and inhalational agent should be kept at minimal to ensure amnesia. I would order a STAT H/H to assess intravascular volume and start volume resuscitation and aggressive inotropic support for cardiac and cerebral perfusion.

Postoperative

Delirium

1. **Patient develops altered mental status in the PACU. How do you differentiate delirium from postoperative cognitive dysfunction?**
   Delirium is characterized by the disturbance of perception, orientation, and psychomotor behavior with a fluctuating clinical course. It usually develops within hours to days. Validation tests of delirium include the Confusion Assessment Method and the Delirium Rating Scale. Postoperative cognitive dysfunction (POCD) typically does not have a clear etiology. The patient presents with fluctuating mental status between postoperative days one and three. The diagnosis of POCD requires baseline preoperative and postoperative neuropsychological testing, with independent risk of advanced age.

2. **The PACU nurse calls you to inform you that the patient's serum glucose is 35 mg/dL. What do you do?**
I would go and assess the patient at the bedside to make sure she is hemodynamically and neurologically stable. After confirming with another finger glucose check, I would start a 5% dextrose intravenous infusion with frequent finger sticks for the next 3 to 4 hours. Transient postoperative hypoglycemia episodes are not unusual in the PACU. This phenomenon is due to a surge of insulin sensitivity secondary to low serum catecholamine levels.

Hypotension

3. **In the PACU, do you anticipate hypertension or hypotension?**
A small percentage of patients remain hypertensive in the postoperative period. If hypertension persists for more than a week, it may suggest an incomplete tumor resection. Most patients after resection of pheochromocytoma experience episodes of hypotension instead. This is a result of persistent preoperative alpha-blockade. Best treatment at this point is probably crystalloid infusion after ruling out potential cardiac issues.

FURTHER READING

Cole M. G. Delirium in elderly patients. *Am J Geriatr Psychiatry* 2004; 12: 7–21.

Fleisher L. E., Beckman J. A., Brown K. A., et al. ACC/AHA 2009 Guidelines on perioperative cardiovascular evaluation and care for noncardiac surgery: executive summary: a report of the American College of Cardiology/American Heart Association Task Force on Practice Guidelines. *Circulation* 2009; 116: 1971–1996.

Lenders J. W., Pacak K., Walther M. M., Linehan W. M., Mannelli M., Friberg P., Keiser H. R., Goldstein D. S., Eisenhofer G. Biochemical diagnosis of pheochromocytoma: which test is best? *JAMA* 2002; 287: 1427–1434.

Orthopedics

10

Shoulder surgery

Sarah J. Madison

STEM 2

A 40 year old male surfer is scheduled for arthroscopic rotator cuff repair at your ambulatory surgery center. He has a history of hypertension and chronic back pain. He has no past surgical history but claims his mother died during surgery from a "high fever."

BP 166/89 mmHg, HR 65 bpm, RR 14, RA SaO_2 99%.

Preoperative

Cardiac

1. **How would you evaluate this patient's cardiac status?**
   I would start with a focused history and physical. In the history, I would ask the patient about any history of heart attack, heart failure, or abnormal rhythms. Given his history of being a surfer, it is likely he lives an active lifestyle but I would still inquire about his physical activity and any ischemic symptoms such as chest pain and shortness of breath. Then I would ask if he had had any diagnostic studies performed such as echocardiogram, exercise tolerance test, or screening EKG. On the physical exam, I would look for any signs of heart failure such as JVD or pedal edema, as well as listen for regularity of rhythm and any murmurs. Finally, I would review any available tests such as EKG or echocardiogram and compare them to previous studies.

2. **How do you know his shoulder pain is not due to cardiac ischemia?**
   This would be determined based on a thorough history and physical as well as a current EKG. If the shoulder pain is reproducible and consistent with an MRI

Rapid Review Anesthesiology Oral Boards, ed. Ruchir Gupta and Minh Chau Joseph Tran. Published by Cambridge University Press. © Cambridge University Press 2013.

lesion, then the pain is most likely stemming from the shoulder. However, if the patient has poor exercise tolerance with signs or symptoms of ischemia, and a remarkable EKG then the shoulder pain is likely cardiac in origin.

Hypertension

3. **How does this patient's history of hypertension affect your anesthetic management?**
The patient's autoregulatory mechanism may be altered. My goal will be to keep his blood pressure within 20% of his baseline (or 30% if the patient is a candidate for an induced hypotensive technique).

4. **The surgeon is requesting "beach chair" positioning. How will this affect your hemodynamic goals?**
I will have to take into account the placement of the noninvasive blood pressure cuff with respect to the patient's head. Cerebral perfusion may be lower than what the blood pressure cuff measures. Also, with venous pooling anticipated in the sitting position, I will have to ensure the patient is well hydrated and have pressors handy during positioning.

5. **Will you agree to a hypotensive technique to optimize visualization during arthroscopy?**
Yes, as long as a recent stress test is normal since I will need to drop the patient's blood pressure within 30% of his baseline.

6. **Other than for surgical exposure, what are some benefits of an induced hypotensive technique?**
It decreases intraoperative blood loss up to 50% and shortens the surgical time by up to one hour.

Malignant hyperthermia

7. **Should this case be done in an ambulatory surgery center or would you insist that it be done in the hospital?**
This patient is a candidate for ambulatory surgery as long as an MH cart is available and all the necessary precautions are taken for this case.

8. **Your resident asks you if you want to delay the case until a muscle biopsy is performed. How do you respond?**
I would not delay the case for a muscle biopsy in this patient because it would not affect my management. Based on the information given, I am going to treat this patient as MH-susceptible and use a nontriggering technique.

9. **What precautions will you take in this patient given his family history?**
First, I will flush out my anesthesia machine with 100% O_2 to remove any residual inhalational agents and remove any triggering agents from the OR

such as succinylcholine. I will make sure I have infusion pumps ready for TIVA. I will have a fully stocked MH cart in the room, and have a team meeting with the nurses and surgeon to discuss the MH protocol and what role each will play. I will have a central line and a-line setup handy and contact the local hospital and ask them if they could reserve an ICU bed for us in the event that this patient develops MH during the case.

Intraoperative

Anesthesia

1. **Will you perform an axillary block for this patient?**
   No. An axillary block will not cover the shoulder. I will perform an interscalene block preoperatively and offer the patient an ambulatory catheter. He may benefit from the opioid-sparing effects of a continuous interscalene catheter infusion.

2. **What is your choice of local anesthetic?**
   If the patient agrees to have a catheter placed, I will use 1.5% mepivacaine for quick onset; I can always re-dose the catheter. If he declines catheter placement, I will use a long-acting local anesthetic like ropivacaine 0.5% for prolonged analgesia. Adding epinephrine, clonidine, or dexamethasone may prolong the block even further.

3. **How will you counsel the patient on postoperative pain management?**
   I would encourage the patient to have an interscalene catheter placed because his chronic opioid use may make it difficult to control the pain with oral opioids alone. A multimodal pain management regimen using a combination of oral opioids and local anesthetics, as well as adjuncts like acetaminophen or NSAIDs, will be more effective than using opioids alone. If he opts for a single-injection block, I will counsel him to start taking his oral opioids before the block wears off.

4. **The patient says to you that his pinky finger doesn't feel numb at all and he thinks the block isn't working. What is your response?**
   This is a normal distribution of an interscalene nerve block. Ulnar sparing (the area of the pinky finger) is common with a properly placed interscalene block.

5. **The surgeon complains that the patient is completely sensate over the anterior deltoid. Your response?**
   The anterior deltoid often receives innervation from the superficial cervical plexus, which is not always blocked with an interscalene. I would test my interscalene block by testing terminal nerve distributions and deltoid strength. If the block were my sole anesthetic, I would perform a superficial cervical plexus block to supplement.

Induction

6. **Let's assume you decided to supplement your regional with a general anesthesia approach. How will you induce this patient?**
    Assuming the patient is NPO, has no other risk factors for aspiration, and has a truly favorable airway exam, I would perform a slow controlled induction using lidocaine, fentanyl, propofol, and rocuronium. I would dose the propofol slowly and carefully to avoid hypotension.

7. **What monitors would you place on this patient?**
    I would place the standard ASA monitors. If the patient shows signs of autonomic instability with induction or positioning, I will have a low threshold for placing an arterial line.

Airway management

8. **The surgeon asks if you can use an LMA for this case. How do you respond?**
    An LMA can be used safely and offers the benefit of spontaneous ventilation in the seated position. However, I will not have access to the patient's airway during the case, and proper seating of an LMA may be challenging to maintain throughout the case. Thus, I would choose to have a secure airway using an endotracheal tube.

9. **Your colleague starts the case for you and places an LMA. Ten minutes into the surgery, your CO_2 machine alarms. You check the circuit and patient and find that the LMA has been dislodged. What is your next step?**
    After alerting the surgeon to the situation, turning on 100% oxygen, and ensuring the patient was adequately deep, I would call for help while attempting to reposition the LMA under the drapes while someone else prepared to mobilize the OR table back to the supine position. If my attempt was unsuccessful, I would place a mask on the patient with 100% O_2 until the table could be repositioned, assisting with ventilation as needed. After an adequate period of preoxygenation and a bolus of propofol, I would secure the patient's airway with an endotracheal tube.

Hypotension

10. **One hour into surgery, your machine alarms again. This time the heart rate is 23 bpm. Blood pressure cuff is cycling. What do you do?**
    I would immediately place the patient on 100% oxygen, check my EKG for a malignant arrhythmia, open the IV wide, alert the surgeon and OR staff, and call for help and a crash cart while feeling for a pulse. If the pulse is weak, I would administer boluses of atropine and epinephrine to raise the HR and BP while someone else starts repositioning the bed to prepare for chest compressions.

11. **What is the mechanism of the bradycardia?**
    There are multiple proposed mechanisms. In a patient undergoing general anesthesia, the most likely is activation of cardioinhibitory mechanoreceptors due to a reduction in preload with a hyperdynamic state (Bezold–Jarisch reflex). Other possibilities include carotid sinus hypersensitivity, orthostasis with venous pooling, and vasovagal response.

12. **Is there anything you could have done to prevent this complication?**
    It has been suggested that epinephrine added to the local anesthetic solution for brachial plexus block may predispose patients to initiate the Bezold–Jarisch reflex. Administration of a beta blocker may be protective; however, actual proof of this mechanism remains elusive.

Postoperative

The remainder of surgery is uneventful. The patient is extubated in the operating room and taken to the recovery room on oxygen facemask.

Pain

1. **The patient complains of pain in the PACU. How will you assess?**
   I would go to the bedside and make sure the vital signs are stable. Next, I will ask the patient about the pain's location, severity, and possible radiation. Next, I would evaluate the block by testing pinprick sensation to determine if the block is providing adequate coverage to the surgical site.

2. **Is there anything you can do to optimize the block?**
   I can check the site to make sure the catheter is in place and no undue pressure is being placed on the extremity. Assuming it was intact, I would administer a bolus of local anesthetic through the interscalene catheter and monitor for any change in pain level.

Dyspnea

3. **Ten minutes after injecting local anesthetic through the interscalene catheter, the patient complains that he is short of breath. How will you assess?**
   I would go to the bedside, assess the patient's vital signs, and make sure he is receiving oxygen by facemask. I would listen to breath sounds bilaterally, visualize chest excursion, and order a chest X-ray.

4. **Breath sounds are diminished on the left. Oxygen saturation is 96%. What is your differential diagnosis?**
   My differential would include pneumothorax and phrenic nerve palsy. Other less likely causes would include unilateral atelectasis, pneumonia, and PE.

Nausea

5. **The PACU nurse calls you to evaluate the patient for nausea. She mentions that the patient's face looks "droopy" and she is worried that he might have had a stroke. How will you assess the patient?**

   First, to evaluate the patient's nausea, I would look at the patient's vital signs, make sure he is receiving oxygen, and ask him about associated symptoms before prescribing an anti-emetic. Then I would examine the patient to determine the etiology of the facial changes, looking specifically for ipsilateral ptosis (Horner's syndrome), which would be a side effect of the block and likely due to the bolus I just administered.

6. **What is your next step in management?**

   Horner's syndrome is an occasional side effect of interscalene block and does not pose risk to the patient. Therefore I would reassure the patient and the nurse that this is a normal finding and the symptoms would resolve in the next several hours.

FURTHER READING

Atchabahian A., Gupta R. (eds.). *The Anesthesia Guide*. New York: McGraw-Hill Publishing, 2013.

Dagli G., Güzeldemir E. M., Acar V. H. The effects and side effects of interscalene brachial plexus block by posterior approach. *Reg Anesth Pain Med* 1998; 23(1):87–91.

Song S. Y., Roh W. S. Hypotensive bradycardic events during shoulder arthroscopic surgery under interscalene brachial plexus blocks. *Korean J Anesthesiol* 2012; 62(3): 209–219.

11

Hip surgery in aortic stenosis

Ruchir Gupta

STEM 1

A 78 year old female presents for emergent ORIF of a hip fracture.

HPI: Patient fell off a chair in her nursing home. The fall was witnessed by a nurse's aide who claimed she did not hit her head and was conscious the entire time.

PMH: Rheumatoid arthritis, hypertension, and aortic stenosis.

EKG: No ST changes, LVH.

PE: HR 111 bpm, BP 98/70 mmHg, RR 23, saturation 95% on 2 L.

Patient has severely limited neck movement.

Lungs are clear to auscultation.

Grade 4/6 systolic ejection murmur.

Labs: Hb 9 g/dL, Hct 27%, platelets 210k.

Preoperative

Hypertension

1. **Are you concerned about her history of HTN?**
   Yes, her history of HTN does concern me. Specifically, I am worried that her HTN may have shifted her autoregulation curve to the right, making it necessary for me to maintain her at a slightly higher MAP to maintain cerebral autoregulation while risking further bleeding into the hip.

Rapid Review Anesthesiology Oral Boards, ed. Ruchir Gupta and Minh Chau Joseph Tran. Published by Cambridge University Press. © Cambridge University Press 2013.

2. **What is the cerebral autoregulation curve? How does HTN affect it?**
   Perfusion to the brain is autoregulated by intrinsic mechanisms over an MAP of 50–150 mmHg. Below and above that range, the perfusion is no longer regulated and becomes dependent on actual blood flow. HTN shifts the curve, such that the range may be higher than the 50–150 mmHg range. Thus, maintaining a MAP of 50 mmHg may cause relative hypotension in a patient who has a history of HTN.

Cardiac status

3. **How does the presence of aortic stenosis (AS) affect your anesthetic management?**
   My primary concern in patients with AS is the development of an MI secondary to inadequate coronary perfusion pressure (CPP). Patients with AS need a high SVR to maintain the coronary perfusion according to the equation: CPP = aortic diastolic pressure – left ventricular end-diastolic pressure. Thus if afterload (aDP) is compromised, CPP will decrease. Therefore, my anesthetic management will be (1) maintaining sinus rhythm because tachycardia not only increases myocardial oxygen demand but also decreases diastolic filling time in the coronary arteries, (2) maintaining adequate preload, (3) maintaining afterload because coronary perfusion pressure (CPP) is afterload dependent according to the equation, and (4) maintaining contractility.

4. **What is the AS transvalvular gradient that would necessitate corrective valvular surgery?**
   50 mmHg.

Intraoperative

Induction and airway

1. **What invasive monitors would you use for this case?**
   I would place a preinduction a-line, CVP, as well as a TEE with a cardiologist available for interpretation.

General vs. regional

2. **Would you perform this case under general anesthesia (GA) or regional anesthesia? Why?**
   I would perform a general anesthetic technique for this case due to the emergent nature of the case, full stomach status, anticipated hemodynamic instability, and history of a difficult airway.

3. **If you had to pick a regional technique for this case, would you decide on a spinal or an epidural?**
   A regional technique is not my first option. But if I had to pick one, I would perform an epidural in this patient since it allows for a greater degree of BP control. The sympathectomy caused by a dilute local anesthetic solution administered slowly through the epidural catheter will not be as great as the sympathectomy caused by a spinal.

Airway

4. **Assuming a GA technique is selected, how would you secure the airway?**
   After a careful airway examination, I would preoxygenate the patient with 100% oxygen, administer GI prophylaxis, and perform an awake fiberoptic intubation with an esmolol drip on standby.

5. **If you selected an awake fiberoptic technique, how would you anesthetize the airway?**
   I would topicalize the airway with nebulized lidocaine and block the superior laryngeal nerve by injecting local anesthetic at the greater cornu of the hyoid bone.

6. **As you introduce the fiberoptic scope into the pharynx, the BP rises to 220/130 mmHg. What are you going to do?**
   I would immediately withdraw the fiberoptic scope, assess the situation while ruling out hypoxia, and recheck the invasive and noninvasive blood pressure readings. If it seems the patient was uncomfortable, I would administer more nebulized lidocaine. If it were due to anxiety, I would titrate in a very small amount of midazolam if reassuring the patient did not work. I would then reintroduce the fiberoptic scope and have an esmolol drip on standby.

Bone cement implantation syndrome

7. **During the operation the patient suddenly becomes hypotensive. What will you do if the BP now reads 75/59 mmHg?**
   I would immediately look at my other vital signs and make sure the patient is not hypoxic, hypocarbic, or in a malignant arrhythmia. I would also recheck the a-line waveform, recycle the noninvasive BP cuff, check an H/H, and look at the TEE for heart chamber filling pressures. After placing the patient on 100% oxygen, I would then pressure bag the IV fluids and begin treatment with a pressor such as epinephrine/ephedrine if bradycardia is present and phenylephrine/norepinephrine if tachycardia is present. I would also communicate with the surgical team and examine the surgical field for active bleeding.

8. **The patient is not hypoxic. You look over at the surgical field and notice that the surgeon is cementing the prosthetic hip joint. How would this affect your further management?**
Methylmethacrylate is a cement used in joint replacements that can cause hypotension usually 30–60 seconds after placement. Treatment involves mainly supportive measures with IV fluids and pressors.

Atrial fibrillation

9. **The patient develops new onset atrial fibrillation with a rapid ventricular response and a corresponding blood pressure of 60/40 mmHg. What would be your immediate actions?**
This is unstable atrial fibrillation. I would put the patient on 100% oxygen, feel for a carotid pulse, confirm the blood pressure readings, call for help, call for a code, and immediately perform synchronized cardioversion. I would also have amiodarone ready. I will send STAT labs including ABG, H/H, electrolytes, cardiac enzymes, and a basic chemistry panel.

Postoperative

Extubation

1. **The surgery is now completed, which took 30 minutes less than anticipated. Are you going to extubate this patient?**
No. This patient developed new onset atrial fibrillation necessitating cardioversion and she suffered multiple bouts of hypotension. In addition, she is a difficult airway and has a diseased myocardium (AS). Thus, I would leave the patient intubated overnight and slowly wean the patient off once her other issues have stabilized. Had this been a routine case and the patient had been completely stable with no adverse events, I would consider extubation.

2. **Assuming you decided to leave the patient intubated, would you use propofol for sedation?**
No, in this patient a propofol infusion can cause life-threatening hypotension given her history of AS. Thus, I would opt for an infusion of midazolam and fentanyl since they are more cardiac stable and provide better hemodynamics.

Postoperative hypertension

3. **Two hours later you are paged to the PACU because the patient's BP has sharply risen to 210/110 mmHg. What are you going to do?**
I would immediately go the patient's bedside and check her vital signs to make sure the patient is not hypoxic, hypercarbic, or in a malignant arrhythmia. Assuming her other vital signs were normal, I would perform a focused history

and physical to determine the etiology and treatment for her hypertension. From the history, I would check the anesthesia record and nurse's notes to see what medications have been given thus far. Because this patient has a history of hypertension, I would also check if she has received her regularly scheduled dose of antihypertensive. From the physical, I would assess if the patient is sedated or is displaying signs of discomfort with the endotracheal tube. I would also see if the patient is sensitive to touch at the operative site. Finally, if everything were negative, I would administer a small bolus of esmolol/ nitroglycerin depending on her heart rate.

4. Would you order any labs?
It is unlikely that any lab work would help me narrow my differential. If I suspected hypoxia or acidosis as a possible cause and my pulse oximeter and/ or EtCO$_2$ monitor were not functioning properly, I would obtain an ABG.

FURTHER READING

Barash P. G., Cullen B. F., Stoelting R. K., Cahalan M., Stock C. M. (eds.). *Clinical Anesthesia*, 6th edn. Philadelphia, PA: Lippincott Williams & Wilkins, 2009.

Herrera A. Valvular heart disease. In: Hines R., Marschall, K. (eds.), *Stoelting's Anesthesia and Co-Existing Disease*, 5th edn. Philadelphia, PA: Churchill Livingstone, 2008.

Miller R. D., Eriksson L. I., Fleisher L. A., Wiener-Kornish J. P., Young W. L. (eds.), *Miller's Anesthesia*, 7th edn. Philadelphia, PA: Churchill Livingstone Elsevier, 2010.

Morgan G. E., Mikhail M. S. *Clinical Anesthesiology*. New York: McGraw-Hill, 2006.

Yao F., Fontes M. L., Malhotra V. (eds.). *Yao and Artusio's Anesthesiology: Problem-Oriented Patient Management*, 7th edn. Philadelphia, PA: Lippincott Williams & Wilkins, 2011.

The burn patient

Ruchir Gupta

STEM 2

A 56 year old, 65 kg female was pulled out of her burning house. She is scheduled for an urgent open reduction and internal fixation of the right ankle. She has a history of HTN and hypercholesterolemia. Vitals: P 105 bpm, BP 90/35 mmHg, RR 24, SaO$_2$ 99% on 2 L supplemental oxygen, T 36.4°C. The patient is stridorous, combative, and has a burn to the face, right upper extremity and torso. She has a 20 g IV in the left arm.

Preoperative

Initial assessment

1. **What are your preoperative concerns in this patient?**
   I have several preoperative concerns in this patient. In terms of airway, I am concerned about her facial injuries, which may distort her anatomy and make her a difficult intubation. Additionally, based on the history given, it is likely she has experienced inhalation injury, which may lead to V/Q mismatch and also CO poisoning. In terms of hemodynamics, burn patients are often severely hypovolemic. Since their capillaries are often leaky, one must be careful to resuscitate them with the appropriate fluid and rate as defined by the Parkland formula. In terms of her GI system, she is at risk for a Curling's ulcer, which may make her full stomach. Finally, I am concerned about her risk of infections because disruption of the skin barrier significantly increases her risk of full-blown sepsis.

Rapid Review Anesthesiology Oral Boards, ed. Ruchir Gupta and Minh Chau Joseph Tran. Published by Cambridge University Press. © Cambridge University Press 2013.

Calculation for percentage burned

2. **The patient has burns to her right upper extremity, torso, and face. What percentage of her body is burned?**

   Thirty-six percent of her body is burned (9% for the upper extremity, 9% for face, and 18% for torso).

3. **If the patient had been a 1 year old, what percentage burn would it be then?**

   Children have different proportions than adults. Thus, for a child the total percent would be 45% (9% for upper extremity, 18% for face, and 18% for torso).

4. **What if in addition to the above, the patient also had a burn injury to her left upper extremity? How would that change the percentage burned?**

   Each upper extremity is 9% in the adult. Thus in addition to her 36%, there would be an additional 9% area burned, for a total of 45%.

CO toxicity

5. **Are you satisfied with this patient's oxygen saturation?**

   No I am not. Based on the information given, it seems very likely that she has suffered inhalation injury and is at risk for carbon monoxide poisoning. Such a condition would not be reflected on a standard pulse oximeter. To ascertain this, a co-oximeter can be used to measure the real oxyhemoglobin saturation.

6. **How does carbon monoxide affect the oxygen hemoglobin dissociation curve?**

   It shifts the curve downward and to the left.

7. **What other conditions shift the oxygen hemoglobin dissociation curve to the left? To the right?**

   The substances that shift the curve to the left are alkalosis, hypothermia, met-HB, fetal Hb, and decreased 2,3-DPG. Conversely, the substances shifting it to the right are acidosis, hyperthermia, and increased 2,3-DPG.

NPO status

8. **Patient ate half a slice of pizza 10 hours ago. Will her burn injuries affect her NPO status?**

   Yes. Patients who experience major burns such as this patient are at risk for developing Curling's ulcers. Thus this patient's gastric volume is greater than that of a normal individual who has been NPO for 10 hours.

Airway evaluation

9. **How are you going to evaluate the patient's airway?**
First, I would perform an external exam, looking for any distorting anatomic features. The presence of stridor in the patient reflects that airway soft tissue swelling has already taken place. Next, I would also assess for any limitations in mouth opening and neck injuries and/or restriction of neck movement.

Intraoperative

Muscle relaxation

1. **Can this patient receive succinylcholine for induction?**
From the standpoint of the burn injuries, it is safe to administer succinylcholine within the first 24 hours. After that time frame, succinylcholine can induce a massive lethal hyperkalemic response.

Airway

2. **How would you secure the airway?**
I would prep and drape the neck for an emergency tracheotomy, have ENT on standby, have the difficult airway cart in the room with different sizes of ETT and LMAs. Then, I would perform a rapid sequence induction with etomidate and succinylcholine after administering GI prophylaxis.

Monitoring

3. **Would you place an arterial line? Where? Pre- or postinduction?**
I would place a preinduction a-line given that she is intravascularly depleted. Because there are burns to the arms, I would place a femoral a-line and use the beat-to-beat monitoring of the BP to assist me during the case to avoid wide fluctuations in BP.

Fluid therapy

4. **Your resident hangs a bottle of albumin during the case to improve the patient's volume status. Is this appropriate?**
No, it is not. Colloids can worsen the hypovolemia by leaking through the capillaries into the extracellular space and increase the oncotic pressure of the extracellular space. This would further result in intravascular volume depletion.

5. **What would be your fluid resuscitation of choice? Why?**
   I would choose a crystalloid solution such as LR in this patient because it is not associated with metabolic acidosis as is the case with NS. Also, leakage of LR through the capillary membranes into the extracellular space will not affect the oncotic pressure the way it would with a colloid.

6. **What is the Parkland formula?**
   The Parkland formula is used to calculate the rate of fluid administration in a burn patient. It is 4 × % BSA burned × weight in kg. Half of this volume should be administered in the first 8 hours, ¼ in the second 8 hours and the remaining ¼ in the last 8 hours.

Postoperative

Extubation criteria

1. **Are you going to extubate this patient?**
   No. This patient is at high risk for airway swelling secondary to her baseline stridor, as well as other complications commonly associated with burns such as sepsis, ARDS, volume overload, and additional surgical procedures. In addition, burns to her torso may impair her ability to take adequate tidal volumes. Thus, I will keep this patient intubated and assess her airway swelling the following day by performing a "leak" test around the ETT. Assuming she has a leak and is able to breathe spontaneously, take adequate tidal volumes without discomfort and her other parameters are normal, I may extubate her in the ICU the following day.

ABG

2. **An ABG performed in the PACU shows: pH 7.30, $PaCO_2$ 55 mmHg, PaO_2 100 mmHg, O_2 saturation 99% on 100% FiO_2. Interpret.**
   This is an uncompensated metabolic acidosis with severe hypoxemia.

3. **Is the PaO_2 adequate? Why or why not?**
   No it isn't. A quick formula to determine an adequate PaO_2 is 5 × FiO_2. Thus in this patient, it should be 5 × 100 for a total of 500 mmHg. This patient has a PaO_2 of only 100 mmHg.

Oliguria

4. **What is the minimum urine output you would want for this patient? Why?**
   Minimum urine output for this patient should be kept at at least 0.5 mg/kg per hour. This is the minimum rate at which metabolic and nitrogenous wastes can be eliminated and normal ranges for electrolytes can be maintained.

Muscle relaxation

5. **The patient returns 2 weeks later for an exploratory laparotomy. The surgeon informs you he will need extreme muscle relaxation for the case. What is your choice for muscle relaxation? Why?**

    I would choose a nondepolarizing muscle agent because a depolarizing agent such as succinylcholine can lead to life-threatening hyperkalemia in the burn patient 24 hours after the burn. This risk is present whenever more than 10–20% of the BSA is burned (this patient has 36% burned). In terms of nondepolarizer I would administer rocuronium in larger than normal doses with re-bolusing as necessary. I will continue to monitor twitches because in any patient with greater than 25% BSA burn injuries, the dose of NDMR can be as high as 3–5 times normal.

FURTHER READING

Atchabahian A., Gupta R. (eds.). *The Anesthesia Guide*. New York: McGraw-Hill Publishing, 2013.

Barash P. G., Cullen B. F., Stoelting R. K., Cahalan M., Stock C. M. (eds.). *Clinical Anesthesia*, 6th edn. Philadelphia, PA: Lippincott Williams & Wilkins, 2009.

Ryan C. M., Schoenfeld D. A., Thorpe W. P., Sheridan R. L., Cassem E. H., Tompkins R. G. Objective estimates of the probability of death from burn injuries. *N Engl J Med* 1998; 338(6): 362–366.

13

Multisystem injury

Raymond Pesso

STEM 1

A 41 year old, 50 kg female presents to the trauma suite for an ORIF of a closed right humerus fracture. Patient was a restrained driver in a motor vehicle accident.

PMH: Hypertension.

PE: VS – HR 110 bpm, BP 90/60 mmHg, RR 24, O_2 saturation 96% on non-rebreather mask.

Airway – Mallampati II.

CV – tachycardic, bruises on left chest.

Respiration – decreased breath sounds on left side.

Abdomen – diffuse tenderness with ecchymosis on the left flank.

Imaging studies: Head CT – negative for any injuries.

Labs: Hb 10.1 g/dL, Plt 240k, WBC 14k cells per mcL.

Preoperative

1. **What is the Glasgow Coma Scale?**
   The Glasgow Coma Scale (GCS) is the most common scoring system used to describe the level of consciousness in a person following a traumatic brain injury. Using three indices (eye opening, verbal response, and motor response), the GCS obtains a combined value between 3 and 15 for any given individual.

Rapid Review Anesthesiology Oral Boards, ed. Ruchir Gupta and Minh Chau Joseph Tran. Published by Cambridge University Press. © Cambridge University Press 2013.

A score below 9 indicates severe brain injury, between 9 and 12 indicates moderate, and 13 or greater indicates minor.

2. **What is the role of an abdominal paracentesis and FAST examination in a trauma patient?**

Abdominal paracentesis is performed when intra-abdominal bleeding is suspected in a hemodynamically unstable patient with a high-risk mechanism of injury. The paracentesis is a means of rapidly diagnosing intra-abdominal injury requiring an exploratory laparotomy.

FAST (focused assessment with sonography for trauma) is a technique to quickly diagnose hemorrhage in a trauma patient using ultrasound. It generally takes <3 min and looks at four different views: RUQ, LUQ, subxiphoid, and suprapubic. The goal is to identify blood accumulation in these areas.

3. **How will you assess this patient's fluid status?**

I will assess the fluid status by performing a focused history and physical examination. From the history, I will review the paramedics' notes as well as the ER notes to see if her vitals have been stable or are gradually getting worse. I will also look at what fluids or blood products she has received since her injury. From the physical exam, I will look for any foci of bleeding and assess her clothes for any blood on them. I will also check any suction canisters to see if they have any blood. I will also look at her mucous membranes, skin turgor, and 2 second capillary refill to assess her current volume status. Finally, I will order a STAT BMP, and ABG to assess for signs of hypovolemia which may manifest as hypernatremia and/or acidosis secondary to lack of tissue perfusion.

4. **Would you order any additional labs for this patient?**

Yes, in addition to the CBC, I would also want a BMP, coagulation profile, ABG, and a type and cross.

Intraoperative

1. **What type of monitoring are you going to use on this patient?**

I would place standard ASA monitors along with an arterial line, a central line, and a Foley catheter.

2. **What kind of IV access would you require?**

For IV access, I would use my central line and also place multiple large bore peripheral IVs.

3. **How would you address the cervical neck concerns of a trauma patient?**

These patients tend to come straight to the OR with a cervical collar in place. It would be prudent for me to speak with the patient as they can verbalize neck pain and even demonstrate neck movements. This would help me determine whether to employ an awake fiberoptic technique or an RSI. If I had negative neck films on A-P view, lateral view, and odontoid view, my concerns would be diminished.

4. **How would you induce anesthesia?**
   Assuming the patient has a normal airway and recognizing that she is a full stomach, I will preoxygenate with 100% O_2, remove the neck collar while having an assistant maintain in-line stabilization, and proceed with a rapid sequence induction. I will induce with etomidate and succinylcholine while applying cricoid pressure. I will also make sure I have the difficult airway cart in the room with various sizes of ETT and LMAs lubed and ready in any emergency situation.

5. **Five minutes after induction the patient's blood pressure drops to 60/30 mmHg while peak airway pressure increases to 25 cmH$_2$O. What is your differential diagnosis?**
   My primary concern would be a tension pneumothorax because of her initial decreased breath sounds on the left. Because she has been in a motor vehicle accident and has ecchymosis over the left flank I would also consider a hemothorax. Other possibilities could be anaphylactic reaction to a recently administered drug, a mainstem intubation, bronchospasm, kinked ETT, ETT obstruction due to a mucus plug, and pulmonary edema.

6. **Patient continues to bleed excessively. A recent ABG shows an Hb of 5.7 g/dL. What is a massive blood transfusion? Would you initiate it at this time? Why?**
   Yes, I would. A massive blood transfusion is defined as replacement of greater than one blood volume in 24 hours or greater than 50% of blood volume in 4 hours. Considering the patient's Hb is 5.7 g/dL and the bleeding is ongoing, the massive transfusion will help maintain tissue perfusion and oxygenation by restoring blood volume, while blood component therapy will help correct any coagulopathic conditions.

7. **What is the ratio of PRBC:FFP:Plt you want to use during a massive blood transfusion?**
   Patients with severe trauma who undergo massive blood replacement and develop secondary coagulopathy have improved survival when the ratio of transfused PRBC:FFP:Plt is close to 1:1:1. Thus, I will start my transfusion based on this guideline and then use my clinical judgment to further guide my therapy.

8. **What are some of the complications associated with a massive blood transfusion?**
   Complications of massive blood transfusion include thrombocytopenia, coagulation factor depletion, hypocalcemia, hyperkalemia, acid/base disturbances, transfusion-related lung injury (TRALI), and acute respiratory distress syndrome (ARDS).

Postoperative

1. **Will you extubate this patient at the end of the operation?**
   Considering that this patient has had a massive blood component replacement, a preexisting lung injury, and anticipated significant third spacing, it is best that the patient remains intubated in the ICU until her fluid status stabilizes and her lab values return to normal.

2. **What are your extubation criteria?**
   I would evaluate the patient for an adequate respiratory drive, respiratory muscle strength, and a cough reflex to clear secretions.

   I would also look at gas exchange, making sure that there is an adequate arterial partial pressure of oxygen with the PaO_2/FiO_2 ratio >300. I would also look for an appropriate pH (pH ≥7.25) and $PaCO_2$ during spontaneous ventilation.

   Other items that are necessary include an RR <35, vital capacity >15 mL/kg, NIF ≥20 cmH$_2$O, tidal volume >5 mL/kg, and a minute ventilation <10 L/min.

3. **You decide to keep the patient intubated and transfer her to the ICU. Patient's temperature is 33.5°C. What are some effects of hypothermia?**
   While mild hypothermia decreases the metabolism of most drugs, wound infection is the most common serious complication, due to impaired immune function and decreased blood flow cutaneously. Hypothermia also reduces platelet function and decreases the activation of the coagulation cascade, while moderate to severe hypothermia can lead to cardiac arrhythmias and death.

   Shivering from hypothermia causes significant increases in oxygen consumption, CO_2 production, and cardiac output.

4. **How will you treat the hypothermia?**
   Hypothermia should be treated with a forced-air warming device, and/or with warming lights or heating blankets which will help raise the patient's body temperature to normal. Heating fluids to near 37°C also helps to prevent hypothermia.

5. **You are paged to the ICU because over the course of several hours, the patient's hemodynamics have deteriorated. CVP is now 22 mmHg, PA 46/25 mmHg, CI 1.5 L/min/m^2 with minimal urine output. What do you suspect is happening? How would you evaluate?**
   I suspect an acute cardiac tamponade and would look for Beck's triad inclusive of hypotension, jugular venous distention, and muffled heart sounds. An echocardiogram would be very useful to look for pericardial fluid and an EKG may show ST segment changes and low voltage QRS complexes. Sometimes a pericardial rub can also be heard with a stethoscope.

6. **How would you treat?**
   I would immediately inform the surgeon, open the IV fluids wide, support the vital signs with dopamine, and prepare this patient for transfer to the OR

for an emergent pericardial window. If the surgeon believes that the patient is a candidate for a bedside pericardiocentesis, I will arrange for IV anesthetic agents as well as resuscitative medicines to be placed next to the patient's bed.

7. **72 hours postoperatively, you notice that the patient has developed progressive hypoxemia. A chest X-ray shows bilateral "white-out" of both lung fields. PaO$_2$ is 64 mmHg on FiO$_2$ of 70%. What is your diagnosis?**

   This patient is most likely in ARDS, which happens to be a form of acute respiratory failure in which the alveolar capillary membrane becomes damaged and more permeable to intravascular fluid. Its diagnosis is usually dependent on signs of acute, refractory hypoxemia, diffuse infiltrates consistent with pulmonary edema, and a pulmonary capillary wedge pressure less than 18 mmHg. These patients usually have a PaO$_2$/FiO$_2$ ratio of less than 200 mmHg.

8. **Will you administer PEEP? How would using PEEP help?**

   Yes. PEEP can help improve oxygenation by preventing alveolar collapse at end-expiration and therefore increase lung volume. This would help improve V/Q matching.

FURTHER READING

Barash P. G., Cullen B. F., Stoelting R. K., Cahalan M., Stock C. M. (eds.). *Clinical Anesthesia*, 6th edn. Philadelphia, PA: Lippincott Williams & Wilkins, 2009.

Morgan G. E., Mikhail M. S. (eds.). *Clinical Anesthesiology*. New York: McGraw-Hill, 2006.

Smith T. C., Marini J. J. Impact of PEEP on lung mechanics and work of breathing in severe airflow obstruction. *J Appl Physiol* 1988; 65(4): 1488–1499.

14

Traumatic brain injury

Ruchir Gupta

STEM 2

A 5'6", 120 kg, 53 year old male presents to the OR for emergent craniotomy. He is somnolent, spontaneously breathing, and speaking incoherently. On physical examination, he has a swollen right arm, ecchymosis into the periorbital area, multiple facial fractures, and several loose teeth. A relative informs staff that the patient has chronic hypertension and bipolar disorder. NS is running through an 18 g IV on the left antecubital arm. VS: HR 129 bpm, BP 180/110 mmHg, RR 28, SaO$_2$ 94% on a non-rebreathable mask. Hb 9.1 mg/dL.

Preoperative

Trauma

1. **The patient has been NPO for at least 8 hours. Is this information helpful?**
   No. Acute trauma victims are assumed to have a full stomach because the stress response from the trauma decreases the parasympathetic nervous system activity and therefore GI motility is diminished. Additionally, it is unclear if this patient has any comorbid conditions that may predispose him to aspiration such as hiatal hernia, diabetic induced gastroparesis, or GERD.

Glascow Coma Scale

2. **As you begin to examine the patient you notice that he opens his eye only to pain, is uttering incomprehensible sounds and is displaying a decorticate response. What is his GCS score?**

Rapid Review Anesthesiology Oral Boards, ed. Ruchir Gupta and Minh Chau Joseph Tran. Published by Cambridge University Press. © Cambridge University Press 2013.

His GCS score is 7. His eye opening to pain is a score of 2, the uttering of incomprehensible sounds is also a 2 and the decorticate response is a score of 3, for a total of 7.

3. **What is meant by a decorticate response?**
A decorticate response is defined as abnormal flexion to painful stimuli.

Intracranial hypertension

4. **What is the difference between epidural versus subdural hematoma?**
There are several differences between an epidural and a subdural hematoma. First, epidural hematomas usually occur from a tear in the midmeningeal artery and collect between the skull and the dura. Subdural hematomas occur after a traumatic brain injury, as seen in this patient, and occur between the dura and subarachnoid layers. In epidural, there is a lucid interval followed by a loss of consciousness whereas in subdural there is no such interval. On a CT an epidural appears as a biconvex shape whereas a subdural appears as a concave shape.

Substance abuse

5. **A toxicology screen done in the ER reveals evidence of cocaine abuse. How does this affect your anesthetic management?**
Cocaine inhibits the reuptake of several substances that are involved in the regulation of the sympathetic nervous system. Chronic abusers will often display labile BP, severe HTN, and possibly difficult vascular access. Acute intoxication can result in ventricular fibrillation, seizures, and catastrophic MI. Thus, I will:
   (1) have a preinduction arterial line to closely monitor the BP and a five-lead EKG to monitor for myocardial ischemia,
   (2) have infusions of nitroprusside and esmolol ready in case I need to rapidly lower the BP,
   (3) make sure I have at least two large bore IVs and, if not, place a central line,
   (4) use only direct acting agents such as phenylephrine and avoid indirect acting agents such as ephedrine because this patient may display an exaggerated response to indirect acting agents,
   (5) use universal precautions for myself and other health care workers because he may have HIV or hepatitis C from IV drug use.

6. **What if the patient was a chronic alcoholic? How would that affect your anesthetic care?**
From a cardiac standpoint, chronic alcoholism can lead to cardiomyopathy. Thus, I will avoid agents that are direct myocardial depressants. From a GI standpoint, cirrhosis or fatty liver may be present depending on severity of the alcoholism. Thus, I will try to avoid drugs that undergo hepatic clearance. I will also avoid any neuraxial techniques because the PT might be elevated.

Also, this patient may have gastritis, so I would use an RSI to secure the airway. From a neuro standpoint, higher MAC values may be needed to keep the patient anesthetized. Thus, I would administer higher than normal MAC values to the patient.

Cervical spine

7. **Can a plain X-ray be used to clear the cervical spine?**
No. An X-ray alone is not sufficient to clear a trauma victim's cervical spine because soft tissue injuries, such as ligament damage, cannot be seen on a plain X-ray.

8. **So how would you clear this patient's cervical spine?**
There are four major components for cervical spine clearance:
    (1) Age >4.
    (2) Absence of cervical tenderness.
    (3) Absence of neurologic deterioration and paresthesias.
    (4) Lack of distracting injuries.
If these conditions were not met, I could use cervical radiographs with A-P views with open-mouth odontoid and lateral views including T1. However, even if these were normal, I would still need a cervical MRI to determine if there is any ligamentous injury that wasn't seen on the X-rays.

Intraoperative

Induction

1. **How will you induce this patient?**
This patient presents as a full stomach and as a potentially difficult airway secondary to his multiple facial fractures that may distort anatomy. In addition, I want to avoid gagging and bucking because that can worsen the ICP in this patient with a head injury. Thus, after prepping and draping the neck for an emergent tracheostomy and having the tracheostomy kit open with ENT on standby, I will perform an RSI with in-line neck stabilization using etomidate and succinylcholine.

2. **What monitors will you place on this patient?**
I will place the standard ASA monitors, central line for fluid management and possible venous air embolism treatment, and an a-line for continuous BP monitoring, serial ABGs, and H/H assessment.

3. **Your resident asks you to use ketamine to maintain spontaneous ventilation in the patient during induction. How do you respond?**
I would inform my resident that ketamine is contraindicated in a patient with increased ICP and can worsen the blood pressure if cocaine is already in his system.

4. **Can you use N$_2$O for maintenance in this patient?**

I would avoid N$_2$O in this patient because I want to avoid any risk of expanding unknown air pockets within the cranium that would worsen the ICP. In addition, I want to maintain this patient on 100% FiO$_2$ given the nature of the injuries. Administration of N$_2$O would inevitably cause me to lower the FiO$_2$.

5. **You determine that this patient has an elevated ICP. What steps can you take to lower the ICP in this patient prior to surgical incision?**

There are several steps that can be taken. First, I could hyperventilate the patient to a PaCO$_2$ of 30 mmHg and elevate the head of the bed 15–30 degrees to promote venous drainage. Next, I would administer mannitol and furosemide as tolerated by the blood pressure, assuming the blood–brain barrier was intact. I could also loosen the neck collar to further promote venous drainage and prevent any venous engorgement of the cranium. Finally, I can consider using a barbiturate to reduce the ICP and decrease the CMRO$_2$.

Blood products

6. **One hour into the case the BP suddenly drops to 70/30 mmHg. What will you do?**

I will immediately look at my vital signs and ensure the patient is not hypoxic, hypercarbic, or in a malignant arrhythmia. I will also recheck the position of my a-line transducer and cycle the NIBP to ensure this is an accurate reading. I will also communicate with the surgeon and look at the surgical field to assess for severe hemorrhaging. Assuming all of my other vital signs are normal, I will open my fluids wide and administer small boluses of a vasopressor such as phenylephrine as a temporizing measure until a definitive diagnosis is made.

7. **You look at your other vital signs and notice that the EtCO$_2$ tracing is at zero. What do you think is going on?**

The highest on my list would be a venous air embolism because hypotension with a loss of EtCO$_2$ in the presence of exposed sinuses places this patient at risk. Other possibilities include a PE, fat embolism, disconnected ETT, myocardial infarction, and a malignant arrhythmia (such as ventricular fibrillation).

Postoperative

Polyuria

1. **You are paged STAT to the PACU because the patient's Na is 124 mEq/L. What is your differential diagnosis?**

Considering the nature of this patient's injury, my differential would be syndrome of inappropriate antidiuretic hormone secretion (SIADH), overhydration, and cerebral salt wasting syndrome (CSWS).

2. **What lab tests would you tell your resident to obtain in order to distinguish CSWS from SIADH?**
I would tell my resident to obtain a urine osmolarity test as well as the hourly urine output for the previous 24 hours. In a patient with SIADH, the urine osmolarity is high, whereas in the CSWS patient, it would be low or normal. In addition, CSWS patients exhibit polyuria whereas SIADH patients will have decreased urine output.

ARDS

3. **On POD #1, the patient develops bilateral infiltrates on CXR and has a PaO_2 of 75 mmHg on 100% FiO_2. What are the criteria for diagnosing ARDS?**
The criteria for diagnosing ARDS are:
   - identifiable etiology
   - acute onset
   - pulmonary artery wedge pressure ≤18 mmHg or absence of clinical evidence of left atrial hypertension
   - bilateral infiltrates on chest X-ray
   - PaO_2/FiO_2 ratio ≤ 200.

4. **What would you call it if the PaO_2/FiO_2 ratio were ≤300 but >200 mmHg?**
In that case, it would be called acute lung injury.

5. **How would you treat the patient under this situation?**
Assuming this is ARDS, treatment is usually supportive with mechanical ventilation, treatment of the etiology with antibiotics if indicated, PEEP to recruit collapsed alveoli, diuretics, and an FiO_2 of 50% or less to prevent oxygen toxicity.

FURTHER READING

Barash P. G., Cullen B. F., Stoelting R. K., Cahalan M., Stock C. M. (eds.). *Clinical Anesthesia*, 6th edn. Philadelphia, PA: Lippincott Williams & Wilkins, 2009.

Miller R. D., Eriksson L. I., Fleisher L. A., Wiener-Kornish J. P., Young W. L. (eds.). *Miller's Anesthesia*, 7th edn. Philadelphia, PA: Churchill Livingstone Elsevier, 2010.

Yao F., Fontes M. L., Malhotra V. (eds.). *Yao and Artusio's Anesthesiology: Problem-Oriented Patient Management*, 7th edn. Philadelphia, PA: Lippincott Williams & Wilkins, 2011.

TURP syndrome

Mark Slomovits

STEM 1

A 76 year old male presents for transurethral resection of the prostate.

PMH: DM, HTN, and hypercholesterolemia.

Meds: Metformin, HCTZ, and simvastatin.

Allergies: Penicillin.

PE: Vitals – BP 112/86 mmHg, RR 16, HR 67 bpm, SaO_2 97% on RA. He has a Mallampati II airway with full cervical range of motion.

The remainder of the physical exam is unremarkable.

Labs: K 3.4 mEq/L, creatinine 1.3 mg/dL.

Preoperative

Assessment of comorbidities

1. **What preoperative information would you want to know before taking this patient to the OR?**
Based on the information given, I would want to know more specific details about this patient's chronic conditions. With respect to his diabetes, I would want to know if it is well controlled, what this patient's HbA1C level is, whether he has any signs or symptoms of any complications from uncontrolled diabetes such as neuropathy, vasculopathy, or nephropathy. In terms of his history of hypertension, I would want to know if it has been well controlled, whether he

Rapid Review Anesthesiology Oral Boards, ed. Ruchir Gupta and Minh Chau Joseph Tran. Published by Cambridge University Press. © Cambridge University Press 2013.

has any complications from long-standing hypertension such as nephropathy or left ventricular hypertrophy. In terms of labs, I would want a CBC to rule out anemia of chronic disease and assess platelet levels, a metabolic panel to determine blood glucose with a BUN/Cr to assess renal function, and a baseline EKG.

2. **You obtain an EKG that reveals left ventricular hypertrophy and Q waves in the lateral leads. How would you proceed?**

The ventricular hypertrophy may be an indication of several conditions, but specific to this patient it may indicate long-standing hypertension. The Q waves are indicative of past cardiac ischemia or an old myocardial infarction and would lead me to assume that the patient has some indolent coronary disease. Furthermore, the presence of coronary disease is worsened in the setting of LVH because of a greater baseline myocardial demand. I would want to compare this EKG to an old one, if available, to see if these changes are new. If they are new, I would insist on the patient undergoing further noninvasive cardiac testing, such as a stress test or an echocardiogram, to ensure the procedure can be performed safely.

3. **Assuming the EKG findings are stable chronic changes, how would you proceed if the platelet count is noted to be 99k and the hemoglobin is 9.8 g/dL?**

I would want to trend the patient's labs with older ones to determine if it is an acute or chronic condition. Given this patient's history of diabetes, this could very well be anemia of chronic disease. Assuming it were chronic, I would type and cross this patient and have blood available before the start of the procedure. If this were acute anemia, I would attempt to determine what the possible cause could be. If the patient's low platelet count were chronic and the patient was otherwise asymptomatic, I would not be concerned. If this were an acute drop, I would want to further investigate and determine the cause.

Laser

4. **The surgeon suggests that he can resect the prostate with reduced bleeding using laser therapy rather than electrocautery. What concerns, if any, would you have with using the laser intraoperatively?**

Laser use in clinical settings is dependent upon their wavelength, energy density, and tissue absorption. Variations in these factors affect the depth and destructiveness of the signal and thus a proper laser would need to be chosen that penetrates the prostatic tissue to the appropriate depth, but also has poor tissue absorption because of the potential for damage to surrounding tissue that is also exposed to the irrigation fluid. There is a risk of fire in the OR if the laser is mishandled, which can be avoided if it is kept in standby mode when not in use. Finally, all personnel (and the patient) should wear proper goggles that are specifically rated to filter out the wavelength of the laser to avoid eye damage.

Intraoperative

Monitoring

1. **What monitors would you want to use for this patient's procedure? Why?**
   In addition to the standard ASA monitors, I would also have an arterial line in place. An arterial line is essential since the patient does have multiple cardiac risk factors and this particular surgery is associated with the risk of massive intravascular volume absorption and subsequent hemodynamic instability.

Regional vs. general anesthesia

2. **Would you perform a general anesthetic or regional technique in this patient?**
   Assuming this patient has no contraindications to a regional such as a coagulopathy or patient refusal, I would choose to perform this case under a spinal anesthetic because I would want an awake patient so that I can assess the mental status during the case.

3. **What are the advantages/disadvantages of each?**
   The benefits of a neuraxial technique in this patient are:
   (1) Ability to monitor mental status in anticipation of possible development of the TURP syndrome/bladder perforation/myocardial infarction.
   (2) Reduced need for systemic opioids for postoperative pain control.
   (3) Avoidance of instrumenting the airway with the associated hemodynamic fluctuations of an induction
   The disadvantages of a regional are:
   (1) Possibility of intraoperative anxiety and awareness in the awake patient.
   (2) Development of a high spinal/epidural necessitating emergent control of airway and maintenance of hemodynamics.
   (3) Inadequate level of blockade (below desired T10).
   With respect to general anesthesia, the benefits are:
   (1) Secure airway.
   (2) Lack of awareness/intraoperative anxiety.
   (3) Ability to ensure proper depth of anesthesia without worrying about level of block.
   The disadvantages are:
   (1) Inability to monitor mental status.
   (2) Increased need for systemic opioids for postoperative pain.
   (3) Necessity of induction with associated hemodynamic fluctuations.

4. **If you choose a neuraxial approach, which type of regional block would you offer? What level of anesthetic blockade would you wish to achieve?**
   I would choose a single shot spinal and attempt a T10 level.

TURP

5. **You perform an uncomplicated bupivacaine spinal anesthetic, achieving a T10 level. Thirty minutes into the procedure the patient complains of nausea and progressively becomes restless and disoriented. What is your differential? What would you do?**

   I would be concerned about cardiac ischemia, cerebral vascular event, hypoxia, pulmonary edema, hyperglycemia, or bladder perforation. However, my immediate concern is for the onset of TURP syndrome. I would immediately look at my vital signs and rule out hypoxia, hypercarbia, hypotension, or a malignant arrhythmia. I would also notify the surgeon of the events and request that they terminate irrigating immediately. I would then control the airway by inducing and intubating the patient and placing him on continuous mechanical ventilation. Finally, I would send off an ABG to evaluate for serum sodium and glucose values.

6. **What would be the properties of an ideal irrigating fluid for a TURP procedure?**

   The ideal irrigating solution should be:
   (1) isotonic – to prevent hemolysis encountered in hypotonic solutions,
   (2) electrically inert – to prevent interference with electrocautery and dissemination of electrical current,
   (3) transparent – to allow proper visualization by the surgeon,
   (4) nontoxic – due to risk of significant systemic absorption.

7. **What is TURP syndrome?**

   TURP syndrome describes a complex of symptoms resulting from acute volume expansion and dilutional hyponatremia manifesting as hypertension (followed by hypotension), refractory bradycardia, and neurologic symptoms that range from vague to severe and may ultimately result in lethargy, tonic clonic seizures, coma, and death.

   Additional information:

   The prostatic urethra is rich in venous sinuses that become exposed during the course of prostatic resection. Since the resection is performed using a cystoscope, the surgical field must be kept clear of resected debris, which is accomplished using continuous fluid irrigation. The exposure of the prostatic sinuses to irrigation fluid (particularly hypotonic fluids) results in systemic absorption, which leads to a dilutional hyponatremia. The absorption volume of irrigating fluid is dependent on the number of open sinuses, the flow rate of the fluid, the hydrostatic pressure of the fluid, the venous pressure at the sinus–irrigant interface, and the duration of the resection. The onset of hyponatremia depends on the rate of the fluid absorption and also on the osmolality of the fluid, where lower osmolality irrigating fluid will contribute to a more rapid development of hyponatremia.

Bladder perforation

8. **Could these symptoms be due to a bladder perforation?**
   Bladder perforation is certainly a possibility because one would still see nausea/vomiting and generalized restlessness as demonstrated with this patient. However, classically there is also shoulder pain from diaphragmatic irritation because most bladder perforations are extraperitoneal.

Hyponatremia

9. **You successfully intubate the patient and initiate mechanical ventilation. An arterial blood gas sample shows: pH 7.46, $PaCO_2$ 22 mmHg, PaO_2 95 mmHg, O_2 saturation 95%, Na 115 mEq/dL, glucose 156 mg/dL. What would be your next step in managing this patient?**
   The hyponatremia is the most pressing concern at this moment and should be corrected by having the surgeon stop all irrigating fluids and by starting an infusion of 3% sodium chloride with the goal of correcting Na at a rate no greater than 0.5 mEq/h. The hypertonic saline should be continued until the symptoms resolve or the serum sodium level reaches 120 mEq/dL, at which point I would switch the infusion to normal saline.

10. **You decide to keep the patient intubated and continue the 3% sodium chloride drip. The vital signs are stable and despite discontinuing all anesthetics the patient is unresponsive. What are you concerned about?**
    My concern would be that a cerebral vascular event or some metabolic disturbance has occurred. The stability of the vital signs argues against any cardiac etiology since hemodynamic instability would be expected.

11. **How would you manage this situation?**
    I would look at the vital signs to make sure the patient is not hypoxic, hypercarbic, hypotensive, or in a malignant arrhythmia. Next, I would also recheck my twitches (paralytic overdose), assess the eyes for pinpoint pupil (opioid overdose), and my end-tidal volatile anesthetic concentration to rule out any anesthetic induced causes. I would also send an arterial blood gas and an electrolyte panel to seek out potential hypo- or hyperglycemia, but especially to evaluate the serum sodium level. Finally, if none of these were the causes, a CT scan of the head may be able to rule in or rule out any cerebral vascular event.

Postoperative

Central pontine myelinolysis

1. **A STAT Na level in the PACU comes back at 128 mEq/dL. It was 115 mEq/dL 2 hours ago. Concerns?**

The rapid rise in serum sodium is concerning as it may result in the patient developing central pontine myelinolysis, a severe demyelinating condition of the brain stem. This state occurs in response to rapid increases in serum osmolality, indirectly measured using serum sodium levels.

Glycine toxicity

2. **The patient recovers and is now awake in the recovery room. He reports blurry vision that progresses to blindness. What do you suspect is occurring?**
In the setting of TURP surgery the onset of blindness is often associated with the use of glycine as an irrigating fluid. Glycine is structurally similar to GABA, and is thus thought to stimulate inhibitory neural pathways, which result in the visual disturbances and may even result in transient blindness.

3. **How would you manage this situation?**
The management of glycine-induced transient blindness is supportive and I would reassure the patient of the transient nature of the condition. Nonetheless, I would ask for an ophthalmologist to evaluate the patient for a more definitive diagnosis.

4. **Do you have any additional concerns with glycine toxicity?**
Transient blindness is suggestive not only of excessive glycine absorption but also of elevated serum ammonia levels since glycine is metabolized into ammonia. The buildup of this by-product can result in altered mental status and even lead to coma until the body is able to adequately clear the metabolite. I would check a serum ammonia level and would want the patient to remain in a monitored setting in case he begins exhibiting any mental status changes.

Oliguria

5. **The nurse reports that there has not been any urine output in the past hour. How would you evaluate the patient?**
The normal urine output for an adult is 0.5 mL/kg per hour and anything less requires evaluation. Low urine output can be broken down into prerenal, intrarenal, and postrenal etiologies and the evaluation should proceed systematically according to these categories. A prerenal etiology relates to a cardiac origin or to hypovolemia. Intrarenal refers to actual kidney failure itself, whether from nephron damage or acute tubular necrosis. Postrenal causes are essentially due to physical obstructions to urine flow whether from tumors, stones, or foreign bodies. The serum and urine electrolytes and creatinine should be checked to calculate the FeNA, or fractional excretion of sodium, which can help identify prerenal causes of low urine output. An ultrasound can be used to evaluate for kidney function as well as for any signs of urine flow obstruction. If there is a urinary catheter, it should be checked for kinks in the tubing or it can be flushed to try to relieve any blockages.

6. **In addition to the low urine output the patient is tachycardic with a heart rate of 112 bpm and reports increasing bladder pressure. How would you manage this situation?**

The findings are most likely indicative of catheter obstruction rather than any intrinsic renal condition. This patient underwent extensive tissue resection within the urethra and is likely forming clots that obstructed the flow of urine. The urinary catheter should be flushed with saline to clear the obstruction and should then be placed on a continuous bladder irrigation. The continuous saline flow prevents the formation of potentially obstructing clots.

FURTHER READING

Atchabahian A., Gupta R. (eds.). *The Anesthesia Guide*. New York: McGraw Hill, 2013.

Barash P. G., Cullen, B. F., Stoelting, R. K., Cahalan, M., Stock, C. M. *Clinical Anesthesia*, 6th edn. Philadelphia, PA: Lippincott Williams & Wilkins, 2009.

Foreign body aspiration

Aimee Gretchen Kakascik

STEM 2

An 18 month, 14 kg male is posted for diagnostic laryngoscopy, bronchoscopy, and foreign body removal. The parents noticed he turned blue and became unresponsive while the family was eating popcorn and watching a movie. 911 was called and emergency service performed CPR. He arrived at the hospital ER after being unresponsive for 15 minutes. The child is currently somnolent with saturations of 93% on a non-rebreathable mask. His blood pressure is 90/54 mmHg, pulse 120 bpm, respirations 32. He has an 18 gauge intraosseous line.

Preoperative

Respiratory

1. **How would you evaluate this patient's respiratory status?**
   I would perform a focused history and physical. From the history, assuming the parents are available I would inquire about the sequence of events leading up to the event. Specifically, was the aspiration witnessed and if so, what was the size and nature of the aspirated foreign material. I would also want to know specifically how long CPR had been performed and whether any emergency medicines such as epinephrine were administered. In addition, I would want to know this patient's baseline respiratory status prior to the event, whether he had any symptoms of a respiratory infection, and any coexisting respiratory diseases such as asthma. From the physical exam, I would look at the child for increased work of breathing (retractions, nasal flaring, tripod posturing,

Rapid Review Anesthesiology Oral Boards, ed. Ruchir Gupta and Minh Chau Joseph Tran. Published by Cambridge University Press. © Cambridge University Press 2013.

drooling, and weakness). I would then examine the airway and auscultate the lungs looking for wheezing and decreased breath sounds on one side. A chest X-ray may indicate decreased lung volumes/atelectasis or hyperaeration of the ipsilateral affected side.

2. What is your differential diagnosis for this patient?

My differential includes foreign body aspiration, esophageal foreign body, croup, reactive airway disease, anaphylactic reaction, epiglottitis, pneumonia, seizure, and cardiac anomaly/arrhythmia.

3. How will you determine the correct diagnosis?

I will auscultate the chest. If there are decreased breath sounds on the right it is most likely a foreign body aspiration. Inspiratory and expiratory radiographic films should be obtained or lateral decubitus in a small child. A mediastinal shift should occur toward the normal side when a foreign body is aspirated.

Vascular access

4. How do you place an intraosseous line?

To place an intraosseous line, I would prep the puncture site with a topical antiseptic, insert either an interosseous needle or a spinal needle into the proximal tibia two fingerbreadths distal to the tibial tuberosity, and advance in a screwlike motion until a loss of resistance was obtained. The needle at this point should be firmly anchored in the bone. Finally I would connect the infusion line and check for any extravasation of fluid.

Airway

5. The child last ate popcorn 3 hours ago. Will you delay the surgery due to his full stomach?

No. While I am concerned about the increased risk for aspiration, the child is also in respiratory distress with a foreign body which may migrate and reobstruct the airway. Further respiratory distress may ensue with irritation and damage from the aspirate.

6. Will you give any premedication to the child?

Yes. I would give an anticholinergic to dry up airway secretions and to minimize the vagal response to bronchoscopy.

Intraoperative

Anesthesia

1. Will you perform a rapid sequence induction on this patient due to the full stomach status?

No. I will perform an inhalational induction and promote spontaneous ventilation to avoid further distal migration of the foreign body which can lead to total airway obstruction or make retrieval technically challenging.

2. **How would you manage if the child aspirated shortly after your induction?**
   I would turn the child's head to the side, suction the oropharynx in a Trendelenburg position, intubate, suction the endotracheal tube, and then ventilate with 100% oxygen.

3. **Assuming the aspiration is now resolved and the ETT is removed at the start of the case, what is your plan for maintaining anesthesia?**
   I would promote spontaneous ventilation and maintain a deep plane of anesthesia with a TIVA technique during the rigid bronchoscopy by the ENT. I would avoid nitrous oxide as it reduces the inspired concentration of oxygen and increases lung volume from air entrapment in the affected lung.

4. **The procedure is proceeding well but the surgeon informs you that the popcorn kernel is too large to fit through the bronchoscope and she must remove it with the forceps and the bronchoscope altogether. She states that she needs the vocal cords to not move. Will you give succinylcholine?**
   I will initially give this patient a propofol bolus to deepen the plane of anesthesia. I will avoid administering succinylcholine to this child since it is not indicated for routine use in the pediatric population. If, after my propofol bolus, the surgeon still does not have the desired relaxation, then I will administer a small dose of rocuronium as a last resort.

5. **The surgeon loses grip of the foreign body while trying to remove it. You are unable to ventilate the patient now. What can be done to improve ventilation?**
   The surgeon should try to remove the foreign body immediately. If she is unable to retrieve it, I would ask the surgeon to push the foreign body distally into the right main bronchus to relieve the total airway obstruction. If this was not successful, I would place the patient into the lateral or prone position in an effort to dislodge the object. Finally, if none of these interventions were successful, the next step would be to place this patient on cardiopulmonary bypass.

Emergence

6. **The kernel is successfully removed. The surgeon states that this was traumatic to the patient's airway and there is much swelling. What can you do to reduce the airway edema?**
   I would administer steroids (dexamethasone 0.5–1.5 mg/kg), humidified oxygen, and nebulized racemic epinephrine.

7. **Will you intubate the patient at the end of the procedure or allow the patient to wake up without an ETT?**
It depends. I would discuss with the surgeon the extent of edema. I would then place a 3.5 cuffed ETT in the patient and measure the airway pressure at which I have an air leak (ideally between 25 and 30 mmHg). If the patient does not have a leak at this pressure, then most likely there is sufficient swelling to cause airway compromise. I would then leave the patient intubated overnight and allow for the swelling to decrease.

8. **It has been 15 minutes and the patient has not awakened from anesthesia. What could be the cause?**
The possible causes for delayed awakening include: hypoxia, hypercapnia, acidosis, hypotension, hypoglycemia, residual anesthesia, inadequate reversal of muscle relaxants, and possible neurologic damage during the arrest.

Postoperative

Postoperative stridor

1. **You decide to extubate the patient and take him to the recovery area. While in recovery the nurse calls you for a breathing treatment because the patient sounds "noisy." What could be the cause?**
The child could be obstructing from soft tissue relaxation, mucosal edema, or bronchospasm from airway irritation of residual foreign body fragments.

2. **How will you assess the patient?**
I will immediately go to the bedside and look at the patient's vital signs. I would also do a focused history and physical, reviewing what medicines were given in the OR and in the PACU, and asking the nurse if the stridor occurred suddenly or gradually. I would also auscultate the lungs while also assessing for increased work of breathing and level of consciousness.

3. **The patient has upper airway stridor; how will you treat?**
I will administer humidified oxygen, steroids, and nebulized racemic epinephrine while monitoring the vital signs, especially the EKG. If the patient has severe obstruction with unstable vital signs and depressed consciousness, I would reintubate with a smaller endotracheal tube and keep him ventilated overnight or until mucosal edema subsides.

4. **What is the mechanism of action of racemic epinephrine?**
It stimulates α-receptors, resulting in vasoconstriction and secondary reduction in mucosal and submucosal edema.

5. **You gave racemic epinephrine an hour ago and now the patient is awake and alert with a room air saturation of 98%. The nurse asks you if the child can be discharged to the ward. What is your response?**

No. I would not discharge the patient from recovery at this point as it has been too soon after epinephrine administration and the patient could have "rebound" edema. Even though he has responded to the racemic epinephrine he should be monitored for at least 3 hours after giving the last dose to make sure "rebound" edema does not occur.

Postoperative nausea

6. **The child vomited in recovery; how will you treat?**

   I would go to the bedside and ensure that the child's vital signs are stable. I will also check electrolytes and fluid status as hypoglycemia and hypovolemia can contribute to nausea. Assuming all of these were normal, I would administer a dose of a 5HT3 antagonist such as ondansetron and also a steroid such as dexamethasone (which may already have been given for airway edema).

7. **The mother says that "Phenergan" was the only thing that helped her nausea after her cesarean section and asks if her son can have it. What is your response?**

   I cannot give promethazine (Phenergan) to her child. There is a US Boxed Warning that respiratory fatalities have been reported in children <2 years of age. Thus, the use of promethazine is contraindicated in this age group. In children ≥2 years, the lowest possible dose should be used and other drugs with respiratory depressant effects should be avoided.

FURTHER READING

Gregory G. A., Andropoulos D. B. (eds.). *Gregory's Pediatric Anesthesia*, 5th edn. Hoboken, NJ: Wiley-Blackwell, 2012; 368, 792–795.

PALS Provider Manual. American Heart Association, 2006; 163–164.

http://media.hsl.washington.edu/media/safranek/fpin/croup-guideline.pdf.

www.fda.gov/Safety/MedWatch/SafetyInformation/SafetyAlertsforHuman MedicalProducts/ucm152554.htm.

17

Tracheoesophageal fistula repair

Peggy Wingard

STEM 1

A 48 hour old, full term infant male weighing 3 kg is brought to the OR for a type C tracheoesophageal fistula (TEF) repair.

HPI: Patient was delivered without complications. Mother of the patient had minimal prenatal care.

PMH: Patient was delivered via vaginal delivery.

PE: Vital signs – HR 135 bpm, RR 30, BP 55/30 mmHg, SaO$_2$ 98% on 0.5 L/min oxygen via NC.

   Lungs – clear to auscultation bilaterally.

   Cardiac – no murmurs heard on heart exam.

X-rays: A blind pouch noted on a lateral view, gas bubbles in the stomach noted on chest/abdomen views.

CXR: No infiltrates seen.

Cardiac echo: Normal cardiac physiology with left-sided aorta arch.

EKG: Sinus tachycardia with T wave inversions in leads V1–V4.

Labs: ABG – pH 7.39, PaCO$_2$ 45 mmHg, PaO$_2$ 85 mmHg; electrolytes are normal with glucose level of 50 mg/dL.

The neonate is brought to the OR with a 24 g IV and an a-line in place.

Rapid Review Anesthesiology Oral Boards, ed. Ruchir Gupta and Minh Chau Joseph Tran. Published by Cambridge University Press. © Cambridge University Press 2013.

Preoperative

TEF

1. **What is meant by a "type C" TEF?**

   A type C TEF has an esophageal atresia (ends blindly in the mediastinum at the level of T2 or T3) with a fistula connecting the distal esophageal pouch to the trachea.

   There are five types of TEF according to the classic Gross classification:

   Type A – esophageal atresia with no connection to the trachea (8%).

   Type B – esophageal atresia with a fistula connecting the proximal esophageal pouch to the trachea (<1%).

   Type C –see above.

   Type D – fistulas connecting the proximal and distal esophageal pouches (2%).

   Type E, the "H-type" fistula – intact esophageal with a fistula connecting to tracheal; there is no esophageal atresia (4%).

   This child has the most common form of a TEF (type C); more than 75% of all TEFs are of this type.

2. **How is a TEF diagnosed?**

   The diagnosis is made at birth when the NGT is unable to be passed beyond 9–10 cm from the mouth and there is increased drooling or when the neonate develops episodes of coughing, choking, and/or cyanosis with the first feeding.

3. **What other congenital abnormalities are associated with TEFs?**

   Associated abnormalities can be remembered by the mnemonic VACTERL. When a child has three or more of the following abnormalities he or she is considered to have VACTERL association.

   V – vertebral/skeletal anomalies (10%),

   A – anal canal defects including anal atresia (14%),

   C – cardiac anomalies including ventricular septal defect, atrial septal defect, tetralogy of Fallot, right-sided aortic arch, and patent ductus arteriosus (30–50%),

   TE – TEF,

   R – renal dysplasia including malposition, hydronephrosis, and ureteral abnormalities (14%),

   L – limb defects including radial aplasia.

   Other associated anomalies include GI involving malrotation of the midgut and duodenal atresia.

Respiratory status

4. What measures can be taken to minimize aspiration preoperatively?
This patient should have a tube (usually a Replogle) placed into his blind-ending esophagus with continual suction and irrigation so that the chances of aspiration are minimized. Also the head should be at a 30° head-up position and kept NPO once the TEF is diagnosed.

5. Would you insist on a gastrostomy tube placement prior to induction?
No. The current thinking is that gastrostomies should no longer be done routinely unless there is concern for severe respiratory issues. The concern for having a gastrostomy in place is that by decompressing the stomach, gas from the trachea bypasses the lungs and exits through the stomach.

Intraoperative

Monitors

1. What monitors will you use for this TEF repair?
Standard ASA monitors, including a pre- and postductal pulse oximeter, a preductal arterial line, and a precordial stethoscope.

Induction/Intubation

2. What are your induction goals for this case?
My primary goal is to adequately ventilate the lungs without ventilating through the fistula and resulting in abdominal distention. Other goals include avoiding hemodynamic instability and aspiration, and maintaining normothermia.

3. How will you secure the airway in this patient?
After performing an inhalational induction with oxygen and sevoflurane, I will place the ETT down the right mainstem (confirming with auscultation) with the bevel of the ETT facing forward and slowly withdraw the ETT until breath sounds become equal bilaterally. My goal is to have the ETT distal to the fistula and proximal to the carina. I will avoid muscle relaxation until the ETT has been confirmed to be in correct position.

Positioning

4. If the patient desaturates during positioning at the start of the case, what is your differential diagnosis?
The ETT could have slipped into the right mainstem, preventing ventilation of the left lung. Alternatively, there could be increased gastric distention causing compromised ventilation. If the patient had a Fogarty catheter in place, I would

be concerned that the catheter has slipped into the trachea, causing partial or total occlusion of the trachea. Other possibilities could include a kinked ETT, a disconnected ETT, or mucus and secretions occluding the ETT.

5. **Had this desaturation occurred in the middle of the case, how would this change your differential diagnosis?**
   In addition to what I previously mentioned, additional causes could be: surgical manipulation of the (soft) trachea causing kinking or displacement of the ETT, surgical compression of vital structures in the mediastinum, and/or compression of the lung resulting in atelectasis.

6. **How will you resolve the desaturation in either situation?**
   I would immediately place the child on 100% oxygen, reassess the other vital signs, confirm placement of the ETT by auscultation with the precordial stethoscope, and listen over the epigastric area for an air leak. I would also call for help, send off an ABG, and notify the surgeon. I would suction the ETT and manually ventilate the patient to assess for compliance as well as provide gentle positive pressure ventilation in the case of atelectasis.

7. **Can a tension pneumoperitoneum cause the desaturation? Mechanism?**
   Yes, it can. If there was increasing gastric distention, the stomach could rupture, leading to a pneumoperitoneum which would impair ventilation.

Postoperative

Extubation

1. **Would you extubate this patient at the end of the case?**
   No. In addition to the increased risk for postoperative apnea in a child less than 60 weeks post-gestational age, I am also concerned about the tension that would be placed at the anastomotic site if this patient were extubated and breathing spontaneously. Instead, I would prefer to have this patient sedated and relaxed until the anastomosis has had a chance to heal (at least 5 days) and ensure adequate pain control.

2. **What postoperative pain management techniques will you use?**
   I will have this patient on a continuous fentanyl infusion of 0.5 to 2 mcg/kg per hour.

Complications of TEF repair

3. **What are the early complications for this kind of surgical repair?**
   Early complications include anastomotic leaks and strictures. Some of the leaks will seal spontaneously and others may require surgical intervention. Strictures can occur at the site of the esophageal anastomosis or the fistula.

4. **What are the late complications for this kind of surgical repair?**

Gastroesophageal reflux is the most common and significant long-standing problem after TEF/EA repair. Other long-term issues include strictures, recurrent aspiration, pneumonia, recurrent lower and upper respiratory infections, reactive airway disease, feeding issues, and oral aversion. Decreased mucociliary clearance also occurs secondary to epithelial cells lacking cilia at the site of the TEF.

Esophageal dysmotility is associated with reduced intrinsic innervation. Tracheomalacia is significant in about 10% of patients and generally identified close to the site of the TEF. Abnormal pulmonary functions include abnormal expiratory flow rates, reduced lung volume, and airway hyperreactivity. There might be associated musculoskeletal malformations secondary to the thoracostomy leading to winged scapula and chest wall asymmetry. Vocal cord paresis has also been reported.

FURTHER READING

Davis P. J., Cladis F. P., Motoyama E. K. (eds.). *Smith's Anesthesia for Infants and Children*, 8th edn. Philadelphia, PA: Mosby, 2011.

Gregory G., Andropoulos D. B. (eds.). *Gregory's Pediatric Anesthesia*, 5th edn. Hoboken, NJ: Blackwell, 2012.

Yao F. F., Artusio, J. F. (eds.). *Yao and Artusio's Anesthesiology: Problem-Oriented Patient Management*, 6th edn. Philadelphia, PA: Lippincott Williams & Wilkins, 2008.

18

Pyloric stenosis

Julio R. Olaya

STEM 2

A 2.9 kg male infant, delivered 21 days ago at 40 weeks gestation, presents with a 48 hour history of non-bilious "projectile vomiting." The child appears lethargic and weak on physical exam. There is a small palpable abdominal mass about 3 cm below the right costal margin with visible peristalsis. His vital signs are: BP 55/36 mmHg, HR 157 bpm, RR 35, T 37°C. Hct = 56%. The patient has an older brother diagnosed with malignant hyperthermia.

Preoperative

Malignant hyperthermia

1. **Does this patient need to have a "halothane caffeine contracture test" to rule out malignant hyperthermia?**
   No. Because this patient has a first degree relative with a known diagnosis of MH, this alone places him at increased risk for developing an MH episode. Thus, the child should be treated with full MH precautions.

Pyloric stenosis

2. **What is your differential diagnosis for this child's presentation?**
   Highest on my differential list would be pyloric stenosis. This patient is presenting the classic signs associated with pyloric stenosis such as male gender, projectile non-bilious vomiting, palpable olive mass with visible peristalsis, and an average age of onset in the range of 5 days to 5 months. Other differential diagnoses include achalasia of the esophagus, duodenal atresia, jejunal/

Rapid Review Anesthesiology Oral Boards, ed. Ruchir Gupta and Minh Chau Joseph Tran. Published by Cambridge University Press. © Cambridge University Press 2013.

ileal atresia, malrotation of the gut, intra-abdominal hernia, and Meckel's diverticulum.

3. **How would you confirm the diagnosis of pyloric stenosis?**
A definitive diagnosis requires an abdominal ultrasound, but a thorough history and physical will reveal classic signs of a palpable mass, projectile vomiting, male gender, and laboratory data consistent with a hypokalemic, hypochloremic metabolic alkalosis.

4. **What electrolyte abnormalities would you expect in this patient?**
I expect to find a hypokalemic, hypochloremic metabolic alkalosis with a compensatory excretion of bicarbonate from the kidneys as well as a compensatory respiratory acidosis. If the electrolyte imbalance is not corrected and the patient continues to dehydrate there will be a shift towards a metabolic acidosis.

Fluids

5. **How would you assess this patient's volume status?**
I would perform a focused history and physical exam. From the history, I would inquire about the frequency and quantity of recent wet diapers, the volume and frequency of the projectile vomit, and whether the patient has received any IV fluids thus far. From the physical, I would assess the vital signs, mucous membranes, presence of sunken fontanels, capillary refill, skin turgor, and mental status.

6. **Your resident suggests using lactated Ringer's for hydration. How do you respond?**
Given the metabolic alkalosis, lactated Ringer's should be avoided since lactate is converted to bicarbonate, thereby worsening the acid–base imbalance. If the patient has a low urine output I would use normal saline until normal diuresis is established, then I would switch to half normal saline, supplementing it with potassium and dextrose.

7. **How do you explain this patient's hematocrit value?**
This child's elevated hematocrit value is most likely due to hemoconcentration as a result of the dehydration and frequent vomiting.

8. **The surgical resident tells you the GI obstruction is a surgical emergency and that the patient must be transferred to the OR immediately. How do you respond?**
I would tell him that this is not a surgical emergency and the patient needs to be adequately volume resuscitated and optimized prior to going to the OR.

Intraoperative

Malignant hyperthermia

1. **How does the child's family history of MH affect your anesthetic management?**
   Given his family history of MH, I would avoid triggering agents like inhalational agents and succinylcholine. I would opt for a TIVA technique, and have the MH cart in the room. I will also transduce an a-line and have proper resuscitation equipment in the room.

Monitoring

2. **Which monitors will you use intraoperatively?**
   I would use the standard ASA monitors (pulse oximeter, EKG, EtCO$_2$, BP cuff, and temperature probe).

Anesthesia and induction

3. **How would you induce the patient?**
   Due to the severe risk for aspiration, the stomach needs to be decompressed either via NG or OG tube in the lateral, supine, and prone positions to remove as much of the gastric contents as possible. After pretreating with atropine (0.02 mg/kg IV), and decompressing the stomach with an OG tube, I would preoxygenate with 100% oxygen, and perform a rapid sequence induction with cricoid pressure to minimize the risk of aspiration. My choice of induction agents are fentanyl, lidocaine, propofol, and rocuronium.

Pediatric airway

4. **What are the key differences between the newborn and adult airways?**
   Newborns have narrow nasal passages, a large tongue, a long and pendulous epiglottis, and a funnel shaped larynx. The position of the neonatal glottis is at the level of C3–4 as opposed to C6 in adults. It is important to note that the narrowest portion in the neonate's airway is 1 cm below the vocal cords (at the level of the cricoid) while it is at the level of the vocal cords in adults.

5. **What size ETT will you use in this child?**
   I would use a 3.0 cuffed ETT for this child. In general, the ETT size for a full term newborn is 3.0 mm, at 6 months it is 3.5 mm, and at 1 year of age it is 4.0 mm. Once the patient is between the ages of 2 and 12 years old, the following guide may be applied:
   Tube length from tip to incisor teeth (cm) would be equal to 11 plus the age in years.
   Tube internal diameter (mm) = 4 + age/4.

Bronchospasm

6. **After intubating the patient you notice difficulty with ventilation. Your resident suggests placing the patient on sevoflurane in order to break the bronchospasm. What are you going to do?**

   I would not use sevoflurane because this patient is susceptible to MH. Instead, I would begin by immediately switching to 100% oxygen, reassessing the other vital signs, deepening my TIVA anesthetic, checking the ETT position, administering a beta-2-agonist like albuterol, and consider giving epinephrine if the symptoms do not improve.

Postoperative

Croup

1. **What are the primary postoperative concerns with this patient?**

   The primary concerns are: continued risk of aspiration, and pulmonary dysfunction including apnea spells secondary to either metabolic alkalosis, hypothermia, or residual anesthesia. I would also be concerned about hypoglycemia from depletion of liver glycogen stores. Finally, postextubation "croup" is a potentially dangerous complication in this age group.

2. **How would you treat postextubation "croup" in this patient?**

   Immediate attention should be paid to a potentially catastrophic postextubation laryngeal edema and the extubation should be carried out by experienced pediatric anesthesiologists.

   Management of croup includes increased inspired oxygen concentration to around 50–60%, nebulized vaponephrine therapy, humidification of inspired gases, and avoidance of excessive narcotics as these may cause respiratory depression.

   Steroids can be helpful and reintubation should be considered if signs of respiratory distress and hypoxia develop.

Postoperative apnea

3. **Is this patient at increased risk for postoperative apnea?**

   Yes. Postoperative respiratory depression occurs commonly in patients with pyloric stenosis. The etiology is unclear but may be due to CSF alkalosis and intraoperative hyperventilation. In addition, infants up to 60 weeks postconceptual age are at increased risk for postoperative apnea. This patient is only 43 weeks.

Postoperative hypoglycemia

4. **Two hours into the patient's PICU stay you notice that the patient has no dextrose in his IV fluid. Are you concerned?**
Yes. Neonates after pylorotomy are at increased risk for postoperative hypoglycemia due to inadequate glycogen stores. Thus, I would immediately switch to dextrose-containing solutions and monitor the patient's blood sugar closely.

FURTHER READING

Hines R. L., Marschall K. E. (eds.). *Stoelting's Anesthesia and Co-Existing Disease.* Philadelphia, PA: Churchill Livingstone, 2008; 599–600.

Kachko L., Simhi E., Freud E., Dlugy E., Katz J. Impact of spinal anesthesia for open pyloromyotomy on operating room time. *J Pediatr Surg* 2009; 44(10): 1942–1946.

Wolfson A. B. *Harwood-Nuss' Clinical Practice of Emergency Medicine*, 5th edn. Philadelphia, PA: Lippincott Williams & Wilkins, 2010.

19

Congenital diaphragmatic hernia

Peggy Wingard

STEM 1

A 7 day old, preterm male weighing 2.5 kg is brought to the OR for repair of a left-sided congenital diaphragmatic hernia (CDH).

PMH: The child was intubated with a 2.5 ETT shortly after birth and placed on low pressure ventilation for respiratory distress and cyanosis. Abdominal ultrasound confirmed the CDH. No other congenital malformations were noted.

PE: Vital signs – BP 50/25 mmHg, RR 60, HR 148 bpm, T 38°C.

Lungs – diminished breath sounds in the right chest, bowel sounds present in the left chest.

Cardiac – no murmurs noted but heart sounds are slightly displaced to the right.

Abdomen – scaphoid appearance.

Labs: ABG – pH 7.26, $PaCO_2$ 55 mmHg and PaO_2 80 mmHg on 30% FiO_2. Hb 16 g/dL, Hct 49%.

Chest X-rays – presence of gas-filled loops of bowel in the left hemi-diaphragm.

The neonate is brought to the OR with a 24 g IV and an a-line.

Rapid Review Anesthesiology Oral Boards, ed. Ruchir Gupta and Minh Chau Joseph Tran. Published by Cambridge University Press. © Cambridge University Press 2013.

Preoperative

Emergent or non-emergent surgery

1. **Is this an emergent surgery? Why or why not?**

   Historically this kind of procedure was considered to be an emergency but current thinking is that the patient must first be medically managed prior to surgery. Medical management of this patient includes stabilizing the cardiorespiratory function by improving oxygenation to have a preductal oxygen saturation >90%, correcting acidosis, reduction of R → L shunt, and increasing pulmonary perfusion (utilizing the least aggressive ventilation possible).

Respiratory/Circulation

2. **Explain the physical exam findings associated with CDH.**

   The physical exam findings I would expect in a child with a CDH include a barrel chest, scaphoid abdomen, bowel sounds on chest auscultation, heart sounds displaced to the right because of the abdominal contents, respiratory distress, and hypoxemia.

3. **Why do patients with CDH develop respiratory distress and cyanosis?**

   Cyanosis results from: (1) atelectasis from the compression of the abdominal contents into the developed lung, (2) pulmonary hypoplasia from the pressure of the herniated abdominal contents resulting in decreased number of alveoli and bronchial generations with medial hyperplasia of pulmonary arterioles, (3) persistent pulmonary hypertension causing increased R → L shunting through a patent foramen ovale and patent ductus arteriosus.

4. **What factors promote R → L shunting in neonates with CDH?**

   The most common factor is pulmonary hypertension since increased pulmonary vascular resistance (PVR) causes deoxygenated blood to be shunted through a patent foramen ovale or a patent ductus arteriosus. Other causes are an imbalance in the production, release, and levels of vasoconstrictors (leukotrienes C4, D4, thromboxane A2, platelet activating factor) and vasodilators (NO, prostacyclin).

5. **How would you treat this patient's pulmonary hypertension?**

   I want to avoid situations that increase PVR such as hypoxia and acidosis. I would have this patient sedated (to minimize stress-induced catecholamine secretion) and paralyzed (to reduce oxygen consumption) and avoid ventilating with 100% oxygen as this will worsen pulmonary hypertension. Other maneuvers include administering NO (a selective pulmonary vasodilator that reduces PVR), HFOV (which improves ventilation while reducing barotrauma), and addition of prostaglandins E1 or D2. ECMO could also be utilized in cases where convention ventilatory maneuvers and HFOV have not worked and there is persistent preductal hypoxemia.

6. **What is the role of permissive hypercapnia in this child?**

It is a technique that is thought to improve the overall survival of neonates with CDH. Small tidal volume and higher levels of PEEP are used to keep the airways open and allow a rise in $PaCO_2$ (60 mmHg). The larger tidal volume needed to maintain normocarbia can cause volutrauma, inducing an inflammatory reaction and release of vasoactive mediators that lead to vasoconstriction and further lung injury (ultimately leading to ARDS). But I do need to be mindful that hypercarbia may worsen PVR.

7. **What is the mechanism of action of nitric oxide (NO)?**

NO causes stimulation of cyclic guanylate cyclase, which increases cyclic GMP. Cyclic GMP activates protein kinases that cause relaxation of vascular smooth muscle.

Intraoperative

Monitors

1. **How are you going to monitor this neonate? If you had a central line where would you place it? Why?**

In addition to the standard ASA monitors and the a-line that is already in place, I will place preductal and postductal saturation monitors. I will place an umbilical central line in this specific patient for several reasons: monitoring of volume status, administration of inotropic agents, administration of blood if needed, and TPN. I would avoid lower extremity central line placement due to inferior vena cava compression with reduction of the hernia. I wish to reserve the neonate's neck veins for possible ECMO therapy. Urine output will be measured with a Foley catheter.

Induction/Intubation/Maintenance

2. **If this patient was not already intubated, how would you secure the airway in this child?**

I would perform an inhalational induction, maintaining spontaneous ventilation, with oxygen and sevoflurane. I will avoid positive pressure ventilation which will further cause respiratory compromise.

3. **What agents will you use for maintenance? Can you use N_2O?**

Provided that the neonate is stable, I will use a combination of O_2/air to maintain oxygen saturation in the low to mid 90s, sevoflurane, fentanyl, and vecuronium. I will use low concentrations of sevoflurane because I am concerned that while these agents produce pulmonary vasodilation and decrease hypoxic pulmonary vasoconstriction (HPV), their effects on SVR are greater than their effects on PVR and may worsen the R → L shunt. I will not use N_2O for several reasons.

I do not want N_2O to diffuse into the abdominal viscera causing additional respiratory compromise and potentially strangulating the herniated bowels.

Ventilation

4. **What are your goals for ventilation? How are you going to achieve them?**
My goals are to avoid barotrauma and provide adequate oxygenation. I will accomplish this by ensuring the airway measurements do not exceed 25–30 cmH$_2$O, a PEEP of 5–7 cmH$_2$O, oxygen saturation of 90–95%, and permissive hypercarbia as tolerated with a pH >7.25.

5. **Will you use 100% FiO$_2$ in this patient if you are worried about hypoxia?**
No. In addition to the risk of the child developing retinopathy of prematurity (ROP), which is seen in patients younger than 44 weeks gestation, I am concerned that 100% oxygen will worsen oxygenation and ventilation as it will recruit additional blood flow to an already less compliant lung and worsen pulmonary hypertension. I will only use 100% oxygen to reverse any acute periods of desaturation and hypoxia.

Decompensation

6. **One hour into the procedure, the patient's saturation drops to 80% while the blood pressure reads 40/20 mmHg. What do you think is happening?**
Top of my differential list is a pneumothorax in the contralateral lung. Other possibilities include: severe pulmonary hypertension, compression of great vessels, acute blood loss, hypovolemia, hypothermia, or allergic reaction to a drug administered.

7. **How will you manage?**
I would immediately look at the other vital signs and make sure the patient is not in a malignant arrhythmia. I will open my fluids and place the patient on 100% oxygen temporarily while I probe for causes. I will inform the surgeon and auscultate the lungs to assess if a pneumothorax (PTX) has occurred. If it has, a needle decompression should be carried out immediately and a chest tube placed by the surgeon. I would also avoid hyperventilation to prevent air leak into the PTX.

8. **(Examiner interrupts) It's not a pneumothorax. What else are you going to do?**
I would then rule out reversible causes. I would instruct the surgeon to relieve compression on the great vessels if they were being surgically compressed. If this were caused by R → L shunting secondary to elevated pulmonary HTN, I would expect a higher pulse oximeter reading on my preductal pulse oximeter than on the postductal pulse oximeter. I would take steps to reduce PVR (NO, hyperventilation) and increase SVR.

9. **How will hypothermia affect this patient?**
    Hypothermia causes an increase in PVR which can lead to an increased R →
    L shunt through the PDA or PFO.

Fluids

10. **Will you give glucose-containing solution during this procedure?**
    Yes. Neonates have decreased glycogen stores and are prone to developing
    hypoglycemia. Maintenance fluids will consist of D5/0.2% NaCl or D5/0.45%
    NaCl at 4 mL/kg per hour. Third space losses will be replaced with LR or 0.9%
    NaCl at 8 mL/kg per hour. Blood loss is replaced in a 1:3 ratio of blood:LR
    and a 1:1 ratio of blood:5% albumin. ABGs, VS, and CVP will guide further
    fluid replacement.

11. **Surgery is now completed. During skin closure the patient's BP drops
    again. What are you going to do?**
    This is most likely due to inferior vena cava compression, resulting in decreased
    cardiac output from diminished venous return. This compression will have
    to be relieved by opening the abdominal cavity and covering the abdominal
    defect temporarily with a Silastic patch.

Postoperative

Extubation

1. **Are you going to extubate this patient at the end of surgery?**
    No. I will leave this patient intubated and maintained on fentanyl and
    vecuronium infusions postoperatively in the NICU. These patients are at high
    risk of various degrees of postoperative pulmonary dysfunctions and I expect
    that the child will further decompensate after a brief honeymoon period.

Decompensation

2. **The child begins to desaturate after 6 hours in the NICU. What
    will you do?**
    I will go by the bedside and ensure that the other vital signs are stable. I will
    then listen to the lungs to make sure that a tension pneumothorax has not
    occurred, obtain an ABG, and assess for pulmonary hypertension.

3. **Would you place this patient on HFOV? ECMO?**
    If this neonate did not respond to maneuvers such as 100% oxygen, and
    hyperventilation from a conventional ventilator, I would place this patient
    on HFOV. If this ventilatory strategy did not work and pharmacological
    intervention did not improve the status, I would consider ECMO.

4. **What is ECMO? Advantages of ECMO? Disadvantages?**

It is a strategy to improve oxygenation/ventilation and myocardial dysfunction. It can be done via venovenous or venoarterial bypass. Venovenous bypass has a double lumen catheter through the internal jugular vein. Blood is removed from and infused into the right atrium through separate ports. Venoarterial bypass has the right atrium cannulated through the internal jugular vein where blood passively flows by gravity into the ECMO circuit, is pumped into a membrane oxygenator and then returned back to the patient through the right common carotid artery into the ascending aorta.

Advantages include elimination or significant reduction of R $\rightarrow$ L shunting through the PDA or PFO and reduction of right ventricular workload (decreased pulmonary blood flow and pressure), pulmonary vasoconstriction (secondary to correction of hypoxia and acidosis by ECMO), and incidence of bronchopulmonary dysplasia (FiO_2 requirements and airway pressure are decreased by ECMO).

Disadvantages include the need for anticoagulation, increased bleeding potential at the surgical and chest tube insertion sites, intracranial hemorrhage, and sepsis.

5. **Are there criteria for going on ECMO?**

Yes, the criteria are: $P(A-a)O_2$ greater than 600 mmHg for more than 6–8 hours, O_2 index of 51 for 5 hours (O_2 index = $FiO_2 \times$ mean airway pressure/PaO_2), gestational age ≥ 34 weeks, weight ≥ 2 kg, and the presence of a reversible disease process.

Outcomes

6. **What are some of the long-term outcomes for these patients?**

These patients may go on to develop reactive airway disease, obstructive lung disease requiring usage of bronchodilators and inhaled steroids, GERD, chest wall deformities, and scoliosis.

FURTHER READING

Davis P. J., Cladis F. P., Motoyama E. K. (eds.) *Smith's Anesthesia for Infants and Children*, 8th edn. Philadelphia, PA: Mosby, 2011.

Gregory G., Andropoulos D. B. (eds.) *Gregory's Pediatric Anesthesia*, 5th edn. Hoboken, NJ: Blackwell, 2012.

Yao F. F., Artusio J. F. (eds.) *Yao and Artusio's Anesthesiology: Problem-Oriented Patient Management*, 6th edn. Philadelphia, PA: Lippincott Williams & Wilkins, 2008.

20

Epiglottitis

Julio R. Olaya

STEM 2

A 2 year old African American boy is brought to the ER for respiratory distress. The child is excessively drooling and leaning forward "to catch his breath." There are substernal retractions along with stridorous respirations. He is complaining of a sore throat. BP 101/80 mmHg, RR 33, HR 130 bpm, O_2 saturation 98% on 2 L oxygen, T 40°C.

Preoperative

Diagnosis

1. **What is the most likely diagnosis in this patient?**
    This patient most likely has acute epiglottitis secondary to an infectious process. Epiglottitis is often bacterial in origin and the most common causative agent is *Haemophilus influenzae* type b.

2. **What are the clinical signs and symptoms of acute epiglottitis?**
    This condition usually begins with complaints of severe sore throat associated with dysphagia and muffled voice. The symptoms rapidly progress and typical pathognomonic signs of dyspnea, drooling, dysphagia, and dysphonia (i.e., the four D's) manifest.

    The illness presents acutely in otherwise healthy children between 2 and 5 years of age with fever as high as 40°C (104°F). In a matter of a few hours the epiglottic inflammation evolves and the child becomes dyspneic. The child usually leans forward and excessive salivation is characteristic as swallowing is difficult. The patient appears anxious and toxic with heavy concentration on breathing.

Rapid Review Anesthesiology Oral Boards, ed. Ruchir Gupta and Minh Chau Joseph Tran. Published by Cambridge University Press. © Cambridge University Press 2013.

3. **Should you wait for culture studies to come back to definitively diagnose epiglottitis?**
   No. Acute epiglottitis is considered an emergency and thus a clinical diagnosis is often sufficient to transfer the patient to the OR for an emergent intubation. If an X-ray had already been completed, it would most likely show a "thumb print" sign on a lateral view.

Volume status

4. **Are you concerned about the child's volume status? How would you assess the degree of dehydration?**
   Yes, I am concerned about his volume status. I would assess his volume status through a focused history from his parents as well as physical examination focusing on skin turgor, capillary refill, heart rate, blood pressure, and mental status.

5. **Would you place an IV in this patient prior to taking him to the OR?**
   No. The placement of an IV in an uncontrolled setting can precipitate a life-threatening episode of laryngospasm.

Selection of anesthetic technique

6. **The father of the patient asks you if you really need to give his child a full-blown general anesthetic (GA) for the intubation. How will you respond?**
   I would tell the father that a general anesthetic is absolutely necessary and that it has many benefits. First, it allows the surgeon to look at the area of the swelling, which would be very uncomfortable for an awake patient. Second, GA would prevent the child from being aware of what is being done to him. Third, GA allows us to maintain a secure airway, deliver oxygen continuously to the patient, and prevent the development of life-threatening hypoxia.

7. **How would you transfer this patient to the OR?**
   Timing is crucial. Once the diagnosis is made, the child will be transported with his parents and a physician with proficiency in airway management (or ENT surgeon) and emergency airway equipment (including a cricothyrotomy kit). I would avoid any kind of upsetting maneuvers like trying to start an IV or separating the child from the parents since crying can potentially trigger respiratory distress and airway obstruction. Nasal prongs or face tent oxygen should be provided and pulse oximetry should be used. Once in the OR, I would have the difficult intubation cart available and an ENT surgeon on standby.

Intraoperative

Airway

1. **How are you going to secure the airway in this patient?**
    I will perform an inhalational induction with sevoflurane and oxygen with the child on a parent's lap in the OR. Once the patient becomes drowsy, I will transfer him sitting up onto the OR table and ask the parent to be escorted from the OR. Once a deep plane of anesthesia has been achieved, an intravenous line is placed, and a careful direct laryngoscopy is performed. I would consider placing an ETT 0.5–1.0 mm smaller than the size I normally use.

2. **Your colleague suggests a rapid sequence induction because the NPO status is unclear. What will you say to him?**
    I will tell my colleague that a slow inhalational induction is the technique of choice because a rapid sequence induction may predispose the patient to severe hypoxia and hypoventilation if intubation is not achieved expeditiously. Once an IV has been established, I would give metoclopramide as a premedication prior to direct laryngoscopy to minimize the risk of aspiration. In terms of NPO status, though it is possible that the patient has not fasted for 8 hours as he normally would had this been an elective case, children with epiglottitis often have difficulty in swallowing secondarily to the pain and discomfort. Thus, it is unlikely that the patient has a full stomach and even if it were it would not alter my management at this time.

3. **How about an awake intubation?**
    No, I would not perform an awake intubation because the risk of losing the airway is very high due to possible adenoidal bleeding, trauma, agitation, laryngospasm, and difficult visualization.

4. **After several intubation attempts, you are still unable to secure the airway. Mask ventilation is becoming progressively more difficult and his saturation is falling. What will you do?**
    I will call for help if I haven't already done so. I would reposition the patient's airway, switch to a different blade, downgrade the size of the ETT, prepare for another direct laryngoscopy attempt while alerting the ENT surgeon for a possible surgical airway, and I would employ jet ventilation to restore the saturation. My attempts to secure the airway using another airway device such as an LMA may be limited due to the swelling of the epiglottis which could lead to further airway obstruction. Thus, in the absence of endotracheal intubation with further patient deterioration, I would want to proceed immediately with a surgical airway if jet ventilation fails.

Postoperative

Extubation

1. **Let's assume you had been able to intubate this patient on your first try. How long would you keep this patient intubated?**
   Usually, it is possible to extubate these patients within 24 to 48 hours.

2. **What will be your criteria to extubate this child?**
   My criteria would be a return of normal body temperature after appropriate antibiotic therapy with either cefazolin, ampicillin with sulbactam, ceftriaxone, or clindamycin, an increased leak around the endotracheal tube, as well as a decrease in erythema and edema.

3. **Would you keep this patient sedated while intubated?**
   Yes. It is important to minimize patient movement and accidental self-extubation.

4. **Is it necessary to admit this patient to the PICU?**
   Yes, it is necessary. This will allow for close supervision of the patient's vital signs, correction of fluid deficits, and adjustments to the ventilator settings.

5. **After 48 hours you decide to extubate the patient. Describe your technique.**
   First, I will ensure that the patient is afebrile with a positive leak test around the ETT. Next, I will transfer the patient to the OR, have ENT on standby with the neck prepped and draped, and induce general anesthesia to allow confirmation of the airway edema resolution by direct visual inspection. Assuming the edema has resolved, I will extubate and continue to monitor closely in the PACU.

FURTHER READING

Bass J. W., Steele R. W., Wiebe R. A. Acute epiglottitis: a surgical emergency. *JAMA* 1974; 229(6): 671–675.

DeSoto H. Epiglottitis and croup in airway obstruction in children. *Anesthesiol Clin N Am* 1998; 16(4): 853–868.

21

Patent ductus arteriosus

Peggy Wingard

STEM 1

A 30 weeks gestation, 1.3 kg male neonate, now 6 days old, presents for repair of a patent ductus arteriosus (PDA).

PMH: Patient was not treated medically for closure of his PDA. Surfactant was administered. Child was intubated shortly after birth with saturations maintained in the mid 80s; he is currently on pressure control ventilation but initially was on HFOV.

PE: Vital signs – BP 45/20 mmHg, HR 178 bpm, RR 40, saturation 87% on 100% O_2.

Lungs – intubated with 3.0 ETT, taped at 8.5 cm at the lips.

Cardiac – S3 present, continuous systolic and diastolic murmur best heard at the left upper sternal border.

Head CT: Small IVH, grade 2.

Echo: PDA of moderate size is present.

Labs: Hb 11 g/dL, Hct 33%, glucose 60 mg/dL.

The neonate is brought to the OR with two peripheral IVs in place.

Rapid Review Anesthesiology Oral Boards, ed. Ruchir Gupta and Minh Chau Joseph Tran. Published by Cambridge University Press. © Cambridge University Press 2013.

Preoperative

Prematurity

1. **What are some concerns with a premature neonate?**
   Besides his PDA and cardiac problems such as shunt reversal, I am concerned about his pulmonary status (compliance, degree of pulmonary hypertension if any), ventilator settings, signs of infection, NEC, electrolyte imbalances including hypo- or hyperglycemia, hypocalcemia, temperature instability, anemia, IVH, and retinopathy of prematurity. In addition, status of TPN and IV access, status of renal and hepatic function (as little as 1 week on parenteral nutrition can cause organ toxicity), and whether the patient has been on chronic steroids which may require steroid coverage in the OR are also of concern.

2. **Your resident asks you why can't the patient receive medical treatment for the PDA closure with indomethacin in place of surgery. How do you respond?**
   Indomethacin is a nonselective cyclo-oxygenase inhibitor that decreases prostaglandin E1 levels and could cause increased intraventricular bleeding in this patient who already has suffered a grade 2 IVH. Thus, indomethacin may not have been a viable option. Additionally, perhaps the PDA is too large to be closed medically, or a trial of indomethacin was administered and the patient did not respond.

3. **Are there any contraindications for using indomethacin in this setting?**
   Yes, the contraindications are intracranial hemorrhage (secondary to platelet dysfunction), renal dysfunction, and hyperbilirubinemia. Adverse side effects of indomethacin include decreased mesenteric, renal, and cerebral blood flow.

Necrotizing enterocolitis (NEC)

4. **Is this neonate at risk for developing NEC? Why?**
   Yes, he is because with a PDA (especially large ones), blood is shunted away from the systemic circulation and towards the pulmonary circulation resulting in decreased abdominal organ perfusion. Since the gut is one of the first organs to be deprived of blood, the child is at risk for developing necrotizing enterocolitis.

PDA

5. **How else can you make the diagnosis of PDA besides the characteristic murmur?**
   During the evaluation of the neonate: bounding pulses, widened pulse pressure, CHF manifested by intercostal retractions, decreased breath sounds, rales, and an S3 sound. Increasing respiratory failure with PaO_2 decreases and $PaCO_2$ increases will require the need for ventilatory support. Echocardiogram will confirm the presence of a PDA.

Intraoperative

Monitors

1. **What monitoring will you use for this neonate? Does the presence of a PDA affect your choice of where to place them?**
   I will use the standard ASA monitors (pulse oximeter, BP cuff, EKG, $EtCO_2$, and rectal temperature probe), a Foley catheter to measure urine output, and a central line if I do not have two well-running PIVs. I will also have an a-line placed in the right upper extremity since clamping of the left subclavian artery may become necessary should the PDA be torn during the procedure. I would place the pulse oximeters in the right hand and lower limb to measure both preductal and postductal readings.

Maintenance

2. **Will you use inhalational agents for maintenance?**
   Inhalation agents, such as sevoflurane, can be used because they are cheap and easily titratable. However, they can cause a decrease in SVR with resulting hypotension. Thus my first choice will be a high-dose fentanyl (30–50 mcg/kg) technique.

3. **What is your target oxygen saturation in this patient? Why?**
   My target oxygen saturation in this patient is between 87% and 95% because this patient is at risk for retinopathy of prematurity. The child's risk factors are (1) prematurity (<32 weeks gestation), (2) mechanical ventilation, (3) respiratory distress, (4) hypoxia, and (5) possible acidosis.

Complication

4. **Midway through the case, the blood pressure suddenly drops and the patient begins to desaturate. What is your differential diagnosis?**
   My differential would be:
   Airway causes: disconnected ETT, kinked or occluded circuit or ETT.
   HD causes: malignant arrhythmia, PE.
   Surgical causes: hemorrhage secondary to tearing of the ductus, ligation of descending aorta or pulmonary artery, lung retraction, pneumothorax.

5. **What will you do?**
   I will quickly evaluate the patient by looking at the VS, EKG, $EtCO_2$, examining the ETT and listening for bilateral breath sounds, looking over the drapes for bleeding, and looking at the suction canisters as well as sponges/lap pads.

Post-ligation

6. What is the vital sign most affected immediately after ligation of the PDA?

Ligation of the PDA may cause systemic hypertension resulting in an increased left ventricular afterload or elevated cerebral perfusion pressure. If the blood pressure rise is not transient, I will administer a vasodilator drug such as nitroprusside or nitroglycerin. If the increased left ventricular afterload causes severe dysfunction of the left ventricle, I will place the patient on an inotropic agent such as dopamine.

Postoperative

Postoperative care

1. Should this patient be on antibiotics postoperatively? For how long?

For 6 months following artificial closure, this neonate should receive spontaneous bacterial endocarditis prophylaxis when undergoing any surgical procedures.

2. Are you going to extubate this neonate if everything went well intraoperatively?

No, I will not extubate this patient. This patient had a relatively large shunt, and is a 31 week premie who initially was on HFOV and came to the OR on a pressure control ventilator. Additionally, he was placed on dopamine in the OR, and has a relatively large incision that may impair ventilation postoperatively due to pain. Thus the patient may benefit from mechanical ventilation for a significant time after surgery.

Had this been a healthy, asymptomatic infant and the procedure went well, I would have considered extubating the neonate in the OR.

The wrong procedure

3. Under what circumstances would you want a PDA to maintain its patency?

When there is an undiagnosed cardiac condition that has ductal-dependent system circulation such as hypoplastic left heart syndrome, aortic valve stenosis, interrupted aortic arch, or coarctation of the aorta. The PDA should be reopened with prostaglandin E1 (0.05–0.1 mcg/kg per min) until the definitive surgical procedure is performed.

Complications

4. What are some complications that are associated postoperatively with PDA ligation?

Depending on the surgical approach, some complications include recurrent laryngeal nerve paralysis, chest wall deformities such as cosmetic defects, scoliosis, and rib fusion. These deformities may be minimized by a percutaneously inserted coil or an occlusion device or doing the procedure via video-assisted thoracoscopic surgery (VATS). Other complications include avoiding retinopathy of prematurity.

FURTHER READING

Davis P. J., Cladis F. P., Motoyama E. K. (eds.). *Smith's Anesthesia for Infants and Children*, 8th edn. Philadelphia, PA: Mosby, 2011.

Gregory G., Andropoulos D. B. (eds.). *Gregory's Pediatric Anesthesia*, 5th edn. Hoboken, NJ: Blackwell, 2012.

Hines R. L., Marschall K. E. (eds.). *Stoelting's Anesthesia and Co-Existing Disease*, 5th edn. Philadelphia, PA: Saunders Elsevier, 2008.

Litman R. *Pediatric Anesthesia, The Requisites in Anesthesiology*. Philadelphia, PA: Mosby, 2004.

22

Tetralogy of Fallot

Ruchir Gupta

STEM 2

A 6 month old female is scheduled for a tetralogy of Fallot repair. The patient has a history of progressively worsening cyanotic episodes since birth. BP 60/30 mmHg, HR 110 bpm, RR 30, O_2 saturation 94% on RA. Hct 55%.

Preoperative

Definition

1. **What is tetralogy of Fallot?**

   Tetralogy of Fallot is a cyanotic heart defect characterized by a constellation of four major anomalies: pulmonic stenosis, VSD, overriding aorta, and right ventricular hypertrophy. Blood is shunted from the right side of the heart to the left, bypassing the pulmonary circulation.

2. **What is the main difference between cyanotic and acyanotic cardiac lesions?**

   In cyanotic cardiac lesions, a fraction of deoxygenated blood from the right side of the heart bypasses the lungs and is shunted into the systemic circulation. Thus, blood ejected from the left ventricle is an admixture of oxygenated and deoxygenated blood. In acyanotic cardiac lesions, oxygenated blood from the left side of the heart is shunted over into the pulmonary circulation. Thus blood that is ejected from the left ventricle into the systemic circulation remains purely oxygenated.

Rapid Review Anesthesiology Oral Boards, ed. Ruchir Gupta and Minh Chau Joseph Tran. Published by Cambridge University Press. © Cambridge University Press 2013.

"Tet spells"

3. **The parents mention that the patient's "Tet spells" have been progressively getting worse. How does a "Tet spell" happen?**
   "Tet spells" are hypercyanotic attacks which occur when there is a relative increase in right-sided heart pressures that further promote right to left intracardiac shunting of deoxygenated blood. An elevated right-sided heart pressure can be caused by an increase in pulmonary vascular resistance, right ventricular outflow obstruction (usually due to a stenotic pulmonic valve), and/ or a decrease in systemic vascular resistance. Normal activities such as crying, feeding, defecating, and exercise can often induce a "Tet spell."

4. **If this child were to develop a "Tet spell" in the holding area, how would you manage the situation without an IV?**
   First, I would call for help and have emergency medications on standby. Next, I would reassess the vital signs while placing the baby on the mother's shoulder with the infant's knees tucked up underneath. This reduces systemic venous return, and increases SVR.

Antibiotic prophylaxis

5. **Do you plan on administering antibiotic prophylaxis for infective endocarditis? Which antibiotic will you administer if there is an IV in place?**
   Yes. I will administer amoxicillin 50 mg/kg IV.

6. **If the child has allergies to penicillin, what is your back-up antibiotic prophylaxis for infective endocarditis treatment?**
   Clindamycin 20 mg/kg IV.

7. **What cardiac conditions require infective endocarditis antibiotic prophylaxis?**
   - Prosthetic cardiac valve or prosthetic material used for cardiac valve repair.
   - History of infective endocarditis.
   - Unrepaired cyanotic congenital heart disease (CHD) (including palliative shunts and conduits).
   - For the first 6 months after completely repairing a congenital heart defect with prosthetic material or device.
   - Repaired CHD with residual defects at the site or adjacent to the site of a prosthetic patch or prosthetic device.
   - Valvulopathy after cardiac transplantation.

Intraoperative

Induction

1. **What are your hemodynamic goals in this patient?**
   The hemodynamic goals in this patient are to avoid conditions that will lower the SVR and/or increase the PVR. Any deviation from baseline parameters will induce a right to left shunting with the development of hypoxemia.

2. **How are you going to induce this patient?**
   After preoxygenating with 100% oxygen, I will perform a smooth IV induction with ketamine (1–2 mg/kg), fentanyl, and rocuronium. The benefit of using ketamine in this child will be that it will maintain or increase the SVR, thereby avoiding a "Tet spell."

3. **Will you use succinylcholine in this patient?**
   No. I want to avoid succinylcholine for two reasons:
   (1) It is not indicated for routine use in the pediatric population as a result of the increased risk for malignant hyperthermia.
   (2) Succinylcholine is associated with histamine release, which can decrease the SVR and promote further right to left shunting of blood.

Onset time of agents

4. **Your resident asks you if a mask induction technique with sevoflurane is preferred for a child with tetralogy of Fallot. How do you respond?**
   I would inform the resident that a mask induction technique is not ideal in this setting since sevoflurane can reduce the SVR in this patient and promote right to left shunting.

5. **How does the presence of a shunt affect the onset time of your IV induction agents in a child with tetralogy of Fallot?**
   The presence of a baseline right to left shunt can speed up the onset time of IV agents since more blood is diverted into the systemic circulation and to end-target vessel-rich organs.

Maintenance

6. **What agents will you use for maintenance?**
   I will want to use a mixture of nitrous oxide, oxygen, and ketamine. Although nitrous oxide is associated with an increase in PVR, these effects are outweighed by the beneficial effect on SVR (no change or modest increase). I would limit the inspired concentration of nitrous oxide to 50% to provide adequate FiO_2 and minimize hypoxia, which can lead to an increase in PVR.

7. **What are the advantages and disadvantages of nitrous oxide for this patient?**

The benefit of nitrous oxide is that it maintains or slightly increases the SVR which will prevent right to left shunting. The disadvantages are that it may also slightly increase PVR, and in order to administer nitrous oxide, the FiO_2 needs to be reduced. A reduced FiO_2 may result in hypoxemia which also results in an increase in PVR.

Blood therapy

8. **Will you have blood in the room for this patient?**

Yes. It is necessary to have blood in the room prior to incision. This is a major surgery with the potential for major bleeding.

Postoperative

Extubation

1. **Will you extubate this patient at the end of the case?**

No. This patient has undergone a major cardiac operation and is also at risk for sudden death due to cardiac causes. Thus, I will want to reduce the work of breathing on this patient by maintaining her on a ventilator overnight and weaning her slowly in the following days.

Hypothermia

2. **Upon arrival to the PICU, the nurse tells you that the patient's temperature is 33°C. What will you do?**

I would place a Bair Hugger on the patient and administer warm fluids through a fluid warmer. I would also place some heated blankets around her head and have the PACU itself warmed.

3. **What are some harmful effects of hypothermia?**

Hypothermia causes a number of deleterious effects including hyperglycemia due to a decrease in plasma insulin, decreased intravascular volume due to cold-induced diuresis, decreased platelet function, and decreased drug metabolism.

Hypoxia

4. **On POD #1 you notice during a routine postoperative visit that the patient's oxygen saturation is 85% on 40% FiO_2. The PICU intern said he turned down the FiO_2 because he was worried about retinopathy of prematurity. How do you respond?**

I would inform the intern that retinopathy of prematurity is only a consideration up to 44 weeks post-gestational age. This patient is already 6 months old and therefore outside of the window during which ROP can appear. I would further inform the intern that this patient needs to have adequate oxygenation because hypoxia will reduce oxygenation to this patient's tissues and may delay healing. The patient's FiO_2 should only be lowered if she is able to maintain adequate oxygen saturation at the lowered FiO_2.

5. **What will you do?**

I will immediately place the patient on 100% O_2, check ETT position, and send an ABG to assess for other respiratory variables to ensure the patient is adequately ventilating and perfusing her tissues.

FURTHER READING

Atchabahian A., Gupta R. (eds.). *The Anesthesia Guide.* New York: McGraw Hill, 2013.

Hines R. L., Marschall K. E. (eds.). *Stoelting's Anesthesia and Co-Existing Disease.* Philadelphia, PA: Churchill Livingstone, 2008.

Stoelting R. K., Miller R. D. *Basics of Anesthesia.* Philadelphia, PA: Churchill Livingstone, 2007.

Intracranial mass

Sergey V. Pisklakov

STEM 1

A 65 year old, 88 kg male is emergently scheduled for a posterior fossa intracranial tumor resection in the sitting position.

HPI: He has a 1 month history of increasing somnolence, headaches, aphasia, gait disturbances, and left-sided weakness.

PMH: Patient has history of chronic hypertension, cigarette smoking, and hypercholesterolemia.

Meds. He is taking HCTZ and Procardia.

PE: VS – BP 196/81 mmHg, pulse 74 bpm, RR 15, O_2 96% on RA.

Neuro – there is moderate bilateral papilledema. Rest of the exam is unremarkable.

CV – RRR.

Lungs – CTA.

EKG: NSR.

Studies: His head CT scan shows a posterior fossa lesion with mass effect.

Labs: Hb 11.8 g/dL.

Rapid Review Anesthesiology Oral Boards, ed. Ruchir Gupta and Minh Chau Joseph Tran. Published by Cambridge University Press. © Cambridge University Press 2013.

Preoperative

Neurologic

1. **Does this patient have increased intracranial pressure (ICP)?**
   Yes. Gradually increasing somnolence, headache, papilledema, and mass effect
   on head CT are markers for increased ICP. The most important thing is to rule
   out Cushing's triad (bradypnea, bradycardia, and hypertension). Other markers
   for increased ICP are nausea, vomiting, headache, and ocular palsies.

2. **What is cerebral perfusion pressure?**
   Cerebral perfusion pressure is mean arterial pressure (MAP) – right atrial
   pressure (RAP) or ICP, whichever is greater.

3. **What premedication would you give to this patient in the holding area to
   alleviate anxiety?**
   Given the fact that this patient is experiencing increased somnolence, I would
   not suspect anxiety to be a major concern. I would refrain from giving any
   anxiolytic at this time. An anxiolytic such as a benzodiazepine carries the risk
   of compounding the somnolence and decreasing the respiration, which will
   increase the CO_2 levels and can lead to possible loss of the airway. Instead, I
   would reassess the patient, looking at the vital signs and perform a focused
   neurologic examination for any acute changes from baseline.

Cardiac

4. **How would you evaluate the patient's elevated blood pressure?**
   Assuming the patient is compliant with his antihypertensive medications, the
   elevated BP is secondary to the elevated ICP. I would evaluate the elevated BP
   by following the ICP trends, serial head CT for the progression of the mass
   effect, and responses to mannitol and furosemide.

5. **How will you manage this patient's BP preoperatively?**
   It is the elevated BP that is permitting adequate cerebral perfusion in response
   to an elevated ICP. Thus, the first step in treating the BP is actually lowering
   the ICP. I would make sure the patient's airway is not obstructed and that he is
   adequately oxygenating and ventilating. Next, I will elevate the patient's head
   30 degrees, have the neurosurgeon drain some CSF, and administer mannitol
   or furosemide. If this is not successful, I will need to place the patient on
   mechanical ventilation and hyperventilate to decrease the $PaCO_2$.

6. **Do you need an echocardiogram in this patient?**
   Yes, if I hear a heart murmur on auscultation. Patients with intracardiac
   shunts such as VSD/ASD, ventriculoatrial shunts, or pulmonary AVMs are
   contraindicated for the sitting position. Thus, I would want a baseline echo to
   rule out these cardiac lesions.

Position

7. **Surgery is to be performed in the sitting position. What are the benefits and drawbacks to a sitting position?**

Benefits of (reasons for) selecting the sitting position:
   (1) Better surgical exposure.
   (2) Less tissue retraction and damage.
   (3) Less bleeding.
   (4) Less cranial nerve damage.
   (5) More complete resection of the lesion.
   (6) Early warning of venous air embolism and brain stem compromise.
   (7) Less facial swelling.
   (8) Ability to observe facial nerve function.

Drawbacks (hazards) to patients in the sitting position:
   (1) Venous air embolism.
   (2) Hypotension.
   (3) Vital sign changes secondary to brain stem manipulation.
   (4) Cranial nerve stimulation (V, VII, X, XI).
   (5) Airway obstruction.
   (6) Excessive neck flexion may cause quadriplegia from cervical spine ischemia.

8. **What are the main advantages of furosemide over mannitol in reducing the ICP?**

Furosemide has several advantages over mannitol:
   (1) Furosemide does not increase cerebral blood volume or ICP.
   (2) It can be used in CHF and/or renal patients.
   (3) It can be used in patients whose blood–brain barrier is compromised.

Intraoperative

Monitors

1. **What kind of monitoring is appropriate for this patient?**

I would use the standard ASA monitors, a preinduction arterial line to monitor hemodynamics closely, a CVP for fluid assessment and for treatment of a venous air embolism (VAE), and possibly a TEE or precordial Doppler ultrasound for detection of a VAE.

2. **What monitors could you use to evaluate cerebral function?**

Several monitors exist, none of which have been consistently shown to improve outcome: EEG, processed EEG, SSEP, transcranial Doppler ultrasound, and cerebral oximetry.

3. **How would you monitor this patient for VAE?**

It is suggested that the precordial Doppler ultrasound in conjunction with expired CO_2 monitoring will fulfill the criteria for monitoring VAE. The TEE is slightly more sensitive in detecting clinical VAE events and is much more sensitive in detecting microbubbles in agitated saline. End-tidal nitrogen concentrations would only be able to detect a catastrophic VAE. In addition, the ventilator and breathing circuit would need to be absolutely free from air contamination. The transcranial Doppler ultrasound will detect air in the cerebral arteries. Its role is currently being evaluated. An esophageal stethoscope will detect a continuous or "mill-wheel" murmur with a severe VAE.

Positioning

4. **What are your concerns for a sitting position?**

My concerns are:

(1) Neck hyperflexion and cervical dislocation.
(2) External pressure on the eyes from the headrest.
(3) Poor visualization, access, and confirmation of the ETT and breathing circuit.
(4) Airway and/or jugular venous compression.
(5) Cerebral ischemia.

Anesthesia plan

5. **What are your main intraoperative considerations for this case?**

The considerations are:

(1) The absolute avoidance of further increases in intracranial pressure.
(2) The provision of intraoperative brain relaxation to facilitate surgical access to the tumor.
(3) Maintaining stable hemodynamics to ensure adequate cerebral perfusion pressure.

6. **What are your main goals during induction? How will you achieve them?**

The main goals during induction of anesthesia are to avoid sudden increases in the intracranial pressure, maintain adequate cerebral perfusion pressure, and avoid cerebral herniation.

I can achieve these goals by having the surgeon preemptively drain CSF through the external ventricular drain and administering mannitol or furosemide prior to induction. Assuming a normal airway, I will preoxygenate with 100% oxygen and perform a rapid sequence induction with lidocaine, fentanyl, etomidate, and rocuronium. I will pay close attention to the preinduction a-line and EKG for VS swings and be prepared to treat them with vasopressors and vasodilators.

7. **Can you use succinylcholine for induction?**

Yes. However, I would be hesitant to administer succinylcholine because of possible further increases, albeit transient, in ICP. If the patient has a reassuring airway, a nondepolarizer such as rocuronium would be a better choice. If, however, this patient was a difficult airway, then the airway would take precedence over the ICP and I would use succinylcholine.

8. **What agents would you choose for maintenance in this patient? Why?**
I would use a balanced technique with fentanyl, isoflurane, and rocuronium. Fentanyl and rocuronium offer the advantage of being cardiac stable, though copious amounts may lead to respiratory depression and delayed awakening. Isoflurane is easily titratable and may offer cerebral protection from the increased ICP.

9. **What are the effects of volatile anesthetics on intracranial pressure? What about intravenous anesthetics?**
Volatile anesthetics increase cerebral blood flow (CBF) and may increase ICP. This effect is significantly exaggerated with persistent hypercarbia. CBF increases linearly with increases in $PaCO_2$ during isoflurane anesthesia and the combination of a volatile anesthetic and hypercarbia can result in higher levels of CBF than either alone. Intravenous drugs, such as propofol, barbiturates, midazolam, and fentanyl, decrease CBF. They also result in a preservation of a linear CBF responsiveness to alterations in $PaCO_2$.

Maintenance

10. **What solution would be the best for intraoperative fluid management?**
All infusions should be prepared with normal saline unless incompatible. Glucose-containing solutions promote cerebral edema and should not be used. Lactated Ringer's solution, although widely used as the replacement fluid in neurosurgical patients, is hypotonic and therefore not as desirable.

11. **As the surgery begins, you notice changes to the somatosensory evoked potential (SSEP). What will you do?**
I will look at my monitors and make sure the patient is not hypoxic, hyper- or hypocarbic, hypotensive, and the MAC value is less than 0.5. Next, I will rule out profuse bleeding as anemia can also cause such changes. I would then inform the surgeon of these changes after ruling out artifacts as the cause with the technician.

12. **The issue is now resolved. After 20 minutes, the surgeon complains of a "tight dura." How can you help?**
Therapeutic maneuvers to improve a "tight brain" are:
    (1) Elevate head slightly to improve venous return.
    (2) Hyperventilate.
    (3) Check oxygenation.
    (4) Check anesthetic agent; possibly need to turn off volatile agent.
    (5) Give propofol to decrease CBV and decrease ICP.
    (6) Give muscle relaxants to decrease ICP and improve venous return.
    (7) Give diuretics to decrease brain edema.

(8) Commence spinal fluid drainage.

(9) Give additional steroids.

(10) Check for intracranial air. If present, pneumocephalus should be aspirated and nitrous oxide discontinued.

13. **Thirty minutes into the case, you notice a sudden drop in $EtCO_2$, hypotension, and tachycardia. What do you think is happening?**
These signs point to a likely venous air embolism.

14. **What are you going to do about this?**
I would:

(1) Immediately inform the surgeon and call for help.

(2) Promptly switch to 100% oxygen.

(4) Have the surgeon irrigate the operative field with saline.

(5) Have the surgeon occlude bone edges with wax to prevent further entrance of air.

(6) Institute gentle compression of the jugular veins.

(7) Aspirate air from the central venous catheter.

(8) Provide hemodynamic support.

Postoperative

Hypertension

1. **The patient was brought to the PACU intubated. One hour later, you notice the BP is 190/100 mmHg. How will you respond?**
I will immediately go to the bedside and confirm that this is an accurate reading while performing a focused neurologic exam and assessing the other vital signs to rule out hypoxia, hypercarbia, or a malignant rhythm. Next, assuming these were normal, I would further assess for the cause such as an elevated ICP, pain, or inadequate sedation. If all of these were normal and the hypertension was an isolated finding, I would infuse a vasodilator such as nitroglycerin.

Peripheral nerve injury

2. **On the third postoperative day, you are told by your resident that the patient is complaining of difficulty dorsiflexing his left foot. How do you respond?**
I would immediately go to the bedside and perform a focused H&P. From the history, I would check the anesthesia record to make sure that the pressure points were adequately padded, specifically areas around the sciatic nerve. I would also ask the patient if he noticed this as soon as he awoke after the surgery or if it started later and whether there is concomitant pain or loss of sensation. From the physical, I would perform a focused neuro exam and assess for any other nerve palsies. I will also evaluate for any signs of inflammation such as rubor, calor, or dolor.

3. **How would you treat this?**

   Assuming this was from a sciatic nerve injury, I would order EMGs and nerve conduction studies and refer the patient for a neurologic consultation. I would also reassure the patient that most of these cases resolve within 6–12 weeks and that he should follow up with a neurologist.

FURTHER READING

Cottrell J. E., Young W. L. (eds.). *Cottrell's Neuroanesthesia*, 5th edn. Elsevier Health Sciences, 2010.

Newfield P., Cottrell J. *Handbook of Neuroanesthesia*, 5th edn. Philadelphia, PA: Lippincott Williams & Wilkins, 2012.

24

Cerebral aneurysm

Sergey V. Pisklakov

STEM 2

A 55 year old, 78 kg female is emergently scheduled for subarachnoid hemorrhage evacuation and intracranial aneurysm clipping. She has a history of a previously diagnosed intracranial aneurysm and was already scheduled for elective intracranial aneurysm clipping. She also has a history of headaches, coronary artery disease, hypertension, cigarette smoking, asthma, and hypercholesterolemia. She is awake and alert, but with a severe headache. Her BP is 176/80 mmHg, pulse 84 bpm, RR 15, O_2 96% on RA. She is currently on metoprolol, Lipitor, and HCTZ. She occasionally takes an albuterol inhaler for her asthma.

Preoperative

Neurologic

1. **How would you evaluate this patient's neurologic status?**
   First, I would perform a history and physical. From the history, I would want to know this patient's baseline neurologic status including possible signs of increased intracranial pressure: somnolence, tiredness, mentation difficulties, worsening headache, and nausea and vomiting. From the physical, I would first assess her vital signs. Specifically, I would be concerned if there was HTN with bradycardia and bradypnea as this can be the Cushing's reflex, which is indicative of elevated ICP. I would also assess global and focal neurologic deficits. Finally, I would look at any imaging studies that are available such as a CT or MRI which may help delineate the size of the hemorrhage.

Rapid Review Anesthesiology Oral Boards, ed. Ruchir Gupta and Minh Chau Joseph Tran. Published by Cambridge University Press. © Cambridge University Press 2013.

2. **What are the normal values of cerebral blood flow?**
   Total cerebral blood flow (CBF) in adults is about 50 mL/100 mg.

3. **What are the determinants of cerebral blood flow?**
   (1) $PaCO_2$. Changes in $PaCO_2$ produce corresponding directional changes in CBF. CBF changes 1 mL/100 g/min for every 1 mmHg change in CO_2 from 40 mmHg. An increase of CO_2 from 40 to 80 mmHg doubles CBF, while a decrease to 20 halves it. Above and below those levels the CBF response plateaus.
   (2) PaO_2. Decreases in PaO_2 do not produce significant increases in CBF until a threshold of 50 mmHg is present.
   (3) pH, neuromediators, and neuromodulators.
   (4) Neurogenic control.
   (5) Temperature.
   (6) Hematocrit.

4. **What is meant by cerebral autoregulation? How does chronic hypertension affect this curve?**
   CBF remains constant between mean arterial pressures of 50 mmHg and 150 mmHg. This is termed cerebral autoregulation. Chronic hypertension shifts the autoregulatory curve to the right such that higher mean arterial pressures are tolerated before CBF becomes pressure-dependent.

5. **The patient complains of a moderate headache and presents with nuchal rigidity. According to the Hunt–Hess classification, what grade is her hemorrhage?**
   According to the Hunt–Hess system, she would be a grade 2 hemorrhage.

Cardiac

6. **How does this patient's history of hypertension affect your anesthetic preparation?**
   Hypertension is a multisystem disease. It is important to know what organ systems are affected in this patient.
   Neuro: Hypertension shifts the cerebral autoregulatory curve to the right. I would avoid lowering the BP to more than 20% from baseline. I would also avoid lowering BP significantly so as to not compromise cerebral perfusion pressure.
   Cardiac: Prolonged hypertension leads to left ventricular hypertrophy and increased myocardial workload. Conversely, even mild hypotension in this patient may have severe consequences because it may impair supply to already diseased myocardium.
   Renal: Hypertension can be a cause of renal failure; thus I would obtain a BUN/Cr to assess renal function.

7. **A preoperative EKG shows T wave flattening with U waves. Are you concerned?**
    I would be less concerned if she does not complain of chest pains or demonstrate dysrhythmias since these EKG abnormalities appear preoperatively in 60% of patients who have subarachnoid hemorrhage (SAH). The EKG alterations are most likely due to increased vagal and sympathetic neural output secondary to SAH. The changes are frequently T wave inversions or flattening, ST segment depression or elevation, U waves, and QT interval prolongation.

8. **What will you do about the EKG findings?**
    I would want to compare the current EKG with a prior one. If these changes are new, I would need to distinguish the etiology as either SAH or cardiac. To rule out a cardiac etiology, I would look for signs and symptoms of an MI such as chest pains, shortness of breath, or diaphoresis.

9. **Will you delay the case?**
    No, because an active SAH is a true surgical emergency.

10. **What labs if any would you want before taking this patient to the OR?**
    I would want a baseline CBC, basic metabolic panel, and a type and cross for 4 units of PRBCs.

Intraoperative

Anesthesia

1. **What are your main hemodynamic goals during induction?**
    My goals during induction are to avoid abrupt changes in BP to ensure adequate coronary and cerebral perfusion while avoiding increasing the BP which could further rupture the aneurysm.

2. **How will you achieve these goals?**
    To achieve these goals I will have in place a preinduction a-line and large bore IVs and plan for a rapid sequence induction with cricoid pressure using etomidate, fentanyl, and succinylcholine. Pressors and vasodilators will be placed on standby to help maintain the hemodynamic equilibrium.

3. **Immediately after induction, the BP suddenly plummets to 70/40 mmHg. What are you going to do?**
    I would check the patient's oxygenation and recycle the BP to make sure this was an accurate reading. I would next look at my EKG tracing to make sure this was not a malignant rhythm. Assuming all of these parameters were normal, I would open my fluids and give a low dose of a vasopressor such as phenylephrine to improve the BP.

Monitors

4. **What kind of monitoring(s) are you going to use in this patient?**

   In addition to the standard ASA monitors (pulse oximeter, BP, EKG, EtCO$_2$, and temperature probe), a preinduction arterial line and Foley catheter are necessary.

5. **What monitors, if any, could you use to evaluate cerebral function? Which is the best?**

   There is no best monitor to evaluate for cerebral function. Several monitors exist, but none of them have been consistently shown to improve outcome: EEG, processed EEG, SSEP, transcranial Doppler, cerebral oximetry, jugular venous O$_2$ saturation, and stump pressures.

6. **What is the role of evoked potential monitoring in this case?**

   Evoked potentials are used to monitor the integrity of specific sensory and motor pathways. Sensory evoked potentials (SEPs) evaluate the functional integrity of ascending sensory pathways, whereas motor evoked potentials (MEPs) test the functional integrity of descending motor pathways. All anesthetics that have been studied influence evoked potentials to some extent. Physiologic factors such as temperature, blood pressure, PaO$_2$, and PaCO$_2$ can substantially alter evoked potentials and must be controlled during intraoperative recording.

7. **You decide to use EEG monitoring. How does this affect your choice of drugs for maintenance?**

   In order to avoid interference with EEG monitoring, I have to make sure I use volatile agents in the value of 0.5 MAC or less.

Blood pressure control

8. **During manipulation of the aneurysm, the surgeon asks you to lower the BP. How do you respond? What is a major conflicting goal with the surgeon's request?**

   I would immediately look at my vital signs, paying close attention to the BP, HR, and EKG. Assuming the patient was otherwise stable, I would gently lower the BP by up to 20% from baseline while paying close attention to any EKG changes. My conflicting goal here is lowering the BP to decrease the transmural pressure while maintaining the coronary perfusion pressure sufficiently to prevent this patient from developing a myocardial infarction.

9. **Is there something you can ask the surgeon to do to decrease the transmural pressure across the aneurysm?**

   Yes. I can ask the surgeon to place a clip on the feeding vessel of the aneurysm.

10. **The surgeon places a temporary clip on the feeding vessel. How would this affect your management?**

Now that the clip is in place, a higher than baseline blood pressure must be maintained to support collateral blood flow to the cerebral tissues.

11. **Can you institute any other measures to offer cerebral protection?**

Yes, I can administer barbiturates which are protective in focal cerebral ischemia because they reduce $CMRO_2$ by reducing cerebral electrical activity. I can also institute hypothermia because doing so will decrease the rate of all metabolic reactions in cerebral tissue. Of course, decreasing the occlusion time and maintaining a higher baseline BP are very efficacious.

Postoperative

Rebleeding and vasospasm

1. **What are your main concerns in the first 12 hours after the operation?**

The most important considerations in SAH are rebleeding and vasospasm.

Rebleeding: Recurrent hemorrhage from an aneurysm is the most devastating complication. It carries a high morbidity and mortality.

Should rebleeding occur, the most important step is to control the ICP by performing an immediate twist drill ventriculostomy and giving mannitol (1.0 g/kg IV). The risk of further hemorrhage is increased after a recurrent hemorrhage. A second bleed is often an indication for immediate surgery.

Vasospasm: Reactive narrowing of the cerebral arterial tree after an SAH occurs in 30% of patients. Treatment for vasospasm includes:

(1) Hypervolemia (PCWP = 18 mmHg; CVP = 12 mmHg).
(2) Hemodilution (Hct in the 30s).
(3) Induced hypertension.

2. **The surgeon asks you to extubate this patient on POD #1. How do you respond?**

My decision to extubate would depend on her intraoperative course. Assuming there has been no rebleeding, the original SAH was small and is evacuated, and cerebral edema is minimal, I would extubate. If, however, there is a high likelihood of cerebral edema and/or there was an intraoperative complication such as rebleeding, I would leave the patient sedated and intubated in the ICU and wait for the cerebral edema to decrease until I can comfortably extubate.

Postoperative hypertension

3. **During a routine postoperative visit, you notice the BP is 190/90 mmHg. How do you respond?**

   I would immediately go to the bedside and confirm that this is an accurate reading while assessing my other vital signs to rule out hypoxia, hypercarbia, or a malignant rhythm including MI. Next, I would perform a focused neurologic and pupillary exam. Assuming these were normal I would further assess for the cause such as anxiety. If no clear etiology could be determined, I might not need to treat because HTN is used for treatment of vasospasm.

Postoperative hyponatremia

4. **The next postoperative day, the patient's serum sodium reads 123 mEq/dL. What are the probable causes?**

   Possible causes include the syndrome of inappropriate antidiuretic hormone (SIADH) and cerebral salt wasting syndrome (CSWS). CSWS occurs as a result of the release of atrial natriuretic peptide. It is characterized by the triad of hyponatremia, volume contraction, and low to normal urine osmolarity. SIADH is characterized by hyponatremia in which the urine is hyperosmolar relative to the plasma. Clinically, SIADH patients are hypervolemic whereas CSWS patients are hypovolemic.

FURTHER READING

Cottrell J. E., Young W. L. (eds.). *Cottrell's Neuroanesthesia*, 5th edn. Elsevier Health Sciences, 2010.

Newfield P., Cottrell J. *Handbook of Neuroanesthesia*, 5th edn. Philadelphia, PA: Lippincott Williams & Wilkins, 2012.

VATS (one lung ventilation)

Ruchir Gupta

STEM 1

A 71 year old, 64 kg, 5'7" female is scheduled for a video-assisted thoracic surgery to remove a right upper lobe carcinoma.

PMH: Asthma, COPD, HTN, hypercholesterolemia, CAD with stents.

PE: BP 152/74 mmHg, pulse 63 bpm, RR 15, RA saturation 93%.

On physical exam, there is digital clubbing and moderate expiratory wheezing.

EKG: NSR, Q waves in II, III, aVF.

Echo: LVEF 48%.

Labs: Hct 54%.

Preoperative

Respiratory function

1. **How would you evaluate this patient's respiratory status?**
   I would start with a focused history and physical. From the history, I would want to know this patient's baseline exercise tolerance, any shortness of breath at rest, compliance with home O_2 therapy, any prior anesthetics or intubations, and any problems weaning off the ventilator. I would also ask if there were any recent changes to her medicines for her COPD. From the physical, I would assess whether she is using any accessory muscle for breathing, any additional

Rapid Review Anesthesiology Oral Boards, ed. Ruchir Gupta and Minh Chau Joseph Tran. Published by Cambridge University Press. © Cambridge University Press 2013.

abnormalities on auscultation besides her wheezing, and whether she is tachypneic. Finally, I would evaluate any studies that may be available to me such as an EKG to assess any right ventricular hypertrophy from her COPD, a baseline chest X-ray and any PFTs.

2. Does this patient need PFTs?

I would not require PFTs in this patient. A focused history and physical can provide me with the information I need: disease severity, possible dependence on home oxygen, response to bronchodilators, exacerbating/alleviating factors, and baseline exercise tolerance.

3. What would you expect her ABG to show?

I would expect a compensated respiratory acidosis with hypoxia. The plasma bicarbonate level would likely be elevated as a compensatory mechanism against the elevated $PaCO_2$.

Cyanosis

4. What do you think of the patient's Hct level and digital clubbing? Are they related?

Yes, they are related because both can occur with chronic hypoxia. Chronic hypoxia can lead to erythrocytosis and pulmonary HTN with subsequent right heart failure. Though the mechanism is unclear, cyanosis can lead to an overgrowth of connective tissue and result in digital clubbing.

Intraoperative

Monitoring

1. How would you monitor this patient?

I would use the standard ASA monitors with a five-lead EKG as well as a preinduction a-line to monitor hemodynamic changes during induction closely. I would also want a Foley catheter.

Epidural catheter placement

2. Assuming this patient stopped clopidogrel 4 days ago, would you place a thoracic epidural for postoperative pain control?

No. Placement of an epidural catheter is contraindicated due to the risk of bleeding. The American Society of Regional Anesthesia and Pain Medicine guidelines require clopidogrel to be held for 7 days, prior to performing an epidural, assuming normal renal and hepatic function. In addition, the case will need to be delayed for an additional 3 days for normal platelet function to resume.

3. **How does clopidogrel work?**
   Clopidogrel is an ADP receptor inhibitor. ADP receptors play an important role in the activation of platelets.

4. **Assuming that she was on aspirin (ASA), instead of clopidogrel, would you place an epidural catheter?**
   Yes. According to the ASRA guidelines, ASA does not increase the risk of a neuraxial hematoma.

Induction

5. **How will you induce this patient?**
   Assuming she has a reassuring airway, I would perform a slow controlled induction using fentanyl, lidocaine, etomidate, and once the ability to ventilate has been established, rocuronium.

Endotracheal tube

6. **What type of endotracheal tube (ETT) will you use?**
   A left-sided DLT is preferable since it provides a greater margin for error in positioning. Ventilation of the RUL can be a challenge with a right-sided DLT due to its proximity to the carina.

7. **What are the absolute indications for DLTs? Relative indications?**
   The absolute indications for DLTs are: bronchopulmonary lavage, bronchopleurocutaneous fistula, lung abscess, bronchial hemorrhage, giant air cyst, or a communicating empyema.
   Relative indications are divided into high priority surgical exposure (pneumonectomy, upper lobectomy, thoracoabdominal aneurysm repair) and low priority surgical exposure (esophageal resection, middle and lower lobectomy).

8. **Your bronchoscope isn't functioning well so you decide to use the "clamp" technique to verify the location of your DLT. Upon inflation of both cuffs and clamping of the tracheal lumen, you hear bilateral breath sounds. What are you going to do?**
   Bilateral breath sounds after clamping of the tracheal lumen suggest that bilateral ventilation is occurring through the bronchial lumen. This can only be possible if the bronchial lumen is in the trachea and not the left bronchus as desired. Thus, I would attempt to push my DLT in further, directing my bronchial lumen into the left main bronchus.

Ventilation

9. **The patient was placed in the lateral decubitus position. What effect does this position have on ventilation?**
   The lateral decubitus position results in greater V/Q mismatch because blood is preferentially directed to the dependent lung while oxygenation is preferentially directed to the nondependent lung.

Hypoxia

10. **Twenty minutes into one lung ventilation (OLV), the patient's oxygen saturation decreases to 93% despite being on 100% oxygen. How do you respond?**
    I would immediately check my other vital signs to make sure the patient is not hypercarbic, hypotensive, or in a malignant arrhythmia, and 100% oxygen would be maintained. Proper DLT positioning would be confirmed by auscultating the chest, while manually providing bag-ventilation. Direct visualization with fiberoptic bronchoscopy would also be used. If that didn't work, I would apply CPAP to the nondependent lung, and then if still unsuccessful add PEEP to the ventilated lung. Finally, if all of these measures failed, I would reinflate the nondependent lung and discuss temporary pulmonary artery clamping.

11. **What if the saturation had dropped to 85% despite your measures?**
    This is a more catastrophic drop in saturation and I would not want to delay restoring the saturation using the aforementioned techniques. Thus, while checking my other vital signs, I would notify the surgeon that I am immediately restoring two lung ventilation.

Massive bleeding

12. **Hypoxemia issues resolve. Thirty minutes later, you notice the patient suddenly develops hypotension with a BP of 72/47 mmHg. What will you do?**
    I would recheck my BP immediately by looking at my arterial-line tracing and recycling the noninvasive blood pressure cuff. I would also check my other vital signs making sure the patient is not hypoxic, hypocarbic, or in a malignant arrhythmia. Assuming these were normal, I would open my fluids wide and communicate with the surgical team, examining the surgical field for active bleeding or other acute event. I would immediately call for blood and administer low doses of a pressor as a temporizing measure.

Postoperative

Extubation

1. **With bleeding under control at the end of the case, would you extubate this patient if the vital signs are stable?**
   No. Given the volume of intraoperative blood transfusion, fluid shifts, and her preoperative COPD status, I would opt to leave this patient intubated in the ICU while her fluid status is improved.

2. **You decide to leave this patient intubated. Your resident asks if you should switch to a single lumen tube (SLT). How do you respond?**
   I would tell him that I will switch to an SLT because it is less bulky and therefore more comfortable for the patient, causes less edema and necrosis, and usually is easier to manage by ICU nurses who may not have experience with DLTs. In addition DLTs have a propensity to reposition more readily than SLTs.

3. **The patient is now in the ICU and an ABG drawn by your resident shows the following: pH 7.30, PaO_2 70 mmHg, $PaCO_2$ 55 mmHg, on 40% FiO_2. Please interpret.**
   This is respiratory acidosis with hypoxemia.

4. **What PaO_2 would you want in this patient with this FiO_2?**
   The ideal PaO_2 on 40% FiO_2 would be 200 mmHg ($FiO_2 \times 5$).

5. **What will you do about this blood gas?**
   I would immediately go to the bedside, place the patient on 100% oxygen, and examine the patient. Specifically, I would evaluate whether the low PaO_2 was due to issues with the ETT or with the patient's ventilation. I would check the position of the ETT, auscultate for bilateral breath sounds, and suction the ETT for any mucus plugs. Assuming these were normal, I would look at the patient's ventilation settings. If she were on SIMV, I would conclude that she is unable to pull adequate tidal volumes on this setting, so I would change her to CMV mode with PEEP and increase her tidal volume as needed. If she were already on CMV, I would look at her ventilation settings and consider increasing her tidal volume and/or respiratory rate.

Postoperative pain control

6. **What are some options for postoperative pain control with this patient?**
   There are several options for pain control in this patient. Assuming the patient is awake and extubated, a PCA would be helpful. The patient also can have regional nerve blocks such as intercostal nerve blocks, paravertebral nerve blocks, cryoneurolysis, and neuraxial techniques. Neuraxial techniques should be used with caution if this patient is on any anticoagulation for her cardiac stents.

Altered mental status

7. **The patient is successfully extubated on POD #1. The ICU nurse pages you because the patient is confused and tachycardic. What is your approach?**
   I would immediately go to the bedside and make sure she is not hypoxic, hypercarbic, hypotensive, or in a malignant arrhythmia. I would then perform a focused history and physical. From the history, I would review the medications that the patient has received in the perioperative period, the medical chart for previously mentioned diagnoses, and the ICU notes to see what medications she has been given, specifically pain medicines because they can cause delirium. The physical examination would include a focused neurological exam, including evaluation of her pupils. Finally, I would order STAT labs including ABG, electrolytes, and glucose. If a stroke seemed possible, a STAT head CT and neurology consult would be obtained.

FURTHER READING

Barash P. G., Cullen B. F., Stoelting R. K., Cahalan M., Stock C. M. (eds.). *Clinical Anesthesia*, 6th edn. Philadelphia, PA: Lippincott Williams & Wilkins, 2009.

Miller R. D., Eriksson L. I., Fleisher L. A., Wiener-Kornish J. P., Young W. L. (eds.). *Miller's Anesthesia*, 7th edn. Philadelphia, PA: Churchill Livingstone Elsevier, 2010.

Yao F., Fontes M. L. & Malhotra V. (eds.). *Yao and Artusio's Anesthesiology: Problem-Oriented Patient Management*, 7th edn. Philadelphia, PA: Lippincott Williams & Wilkins, 2011.

Mediastinal mass

Stanley Yuan and Joseph Marino

A 32 year old male presents for biopsy of a mediastinal mass. He complains of difficulty swallowing for the past several weeks. His past medical history is significant for severe asthma. His medications include albuterol, pyridostigmine, and Advair. VS: HR 76 bpm, BP 112/67 mmHg, RR 14, O_2 saturation 96% on RA. Hb 11.4 g/dL, Plt 290k.

Preoperative

Airway

1. **How would you evaluate the extent of this patient's mediastinal mass?**
   I would perform a full history and physical. I would want to know how long this patient has had dysphagia, progression of the symptoms, and aggravating or alleviating factors. I would also inquire about any signs of superior vena cava syndrome such as headache, confusion, and altered mental status. From the physical exam, I would look for any gross deviations in the oropharynx and palpable masses in the neck. I would also look for signs of SVC syndrome such as facial cyanosis, venous distention of the neck or arm, and any edema of the upper extremity. Finally, imaging studies such as a CT or MRI are valuable to determine the location and size of the mass as well as the degree of tracheal deviation.

2. **How does the presence of a mediastinal mass affect your anesthetic plan?**
   A mediastinal mass can result in airway and cardiovascular collapse. Depending on size and location, most of these cases are not amenable to local anesthesia. The primary goal of general anesthesia is to secure the airway while keeping the patient spontaneously breathing.

Rapid Review Anesthesiology Oral Boards, ed. Ruchir Gupta and Minh Chau Joseph Tran. Published by Cambridge University Press. © Cambridge University Press 2013.

3. **Are flow volume loops essential as part of the preoperative assessment? What about an echocardiogram?**

No. Flow volume loops have been shown to correlate poorly to the degree of airway obstruction and have not been useful in managing these types of patients. The most useful information comes from the history and physical as well as pertinent imaging studies. An echocardiogram would be indicated if there were additional symptoms such as shortness of breath or congestive heart failure. In the absence of these symptoms, I would not rush to order an echocardiogram at this time as it will not affect my management.

Asthma

4. **How would you assess this patient's asthma?**

I would first assess this patient's asthma by performing a focused history and physical. From the history, I would elicit how long the patient has had asthma, whether he has ever had to go to the emergency department for an exacerbation, and whether he has had any hospitalizations or intubations as a result of the asthma. I would also want to know the aggravating/alleviating factors, degree of improvement from the inhaler, and any complications with past anesthetics. I would also inquire about any recent chest colds or upper respiratory infections. From the physical, I would assess to see if this patient is breathing comfortably, whether any accessory muscle use is occurring, and whether any wheezes or rhonchi are present. Finally, I would review any imaging studies such as a chest X-ray if available.

Endocrine status

5. **Why is this patient on pyridostigmine?**

As an anticholinesterase inhibitor, pyridostigmine is normally given to patients with myasthenia gravis since it is an autoimmune disease where circulating antibodies bind to acetylcholine receptors, rendering them inactive. Pyridostigmine increases the concentration of circulating acetylcholine molecules, thereby increasing the probability that acetylcholine will bind to the receptors.

6. **How does pyridostigmine impact your anesthetic planning for this case?**

The patient's chronic use of pyridostigmine may interfere with the ability to reverse this patient's paralysis. Thus, the patient may remain paralyzed for a prolonged period of time, necessitating the use of postoperative ventilation.

7. **Would you continue the pyridostigmine on the day of surgery?**

Yes. I would tell the patient to continue his medication on the day of surgery and also inform him of the potential necessity of postoperative ventilator support.

Intraoperative

Induction

1. **What intraoperative monitors would you use for induction?**
   In addition to the standard ASA monitors, I would like to place an arterial line in the right radial artery to evaluate innominate artery compression during mediastinoscopy. I would want to have one pulse oximeter in the right upper extremity to diagnose right innominate artery compression and one in the lower extremity in case I lost my pulse oximeter tracing in the upper extremity during the procedure. For a large mediastinal mass, I would also consider placing bilateral femoral lines so that in cases of life-threatening airway collapse, cardiopulmonary bypass can be initiated.

2. **How would you induce this patient?**
   A discussion with the surgeon is needed to confirm that a rigid bronchoscope is immediately available and a sternal saw if life-threatening airway compromise occurs. I would preserve spontaneous ventilation and perform an awake fiberoptic intubation by topicalizing the airway using viscous lidocaine spray. If needed, I would titrate ketamine for its bronchodilatory effect and ability to maintain spontaneous ventilation.

3. **The patient refuses an awake fiberoptic intubation. Now what?**
   I would have a detailed discussion with the patient about the risks involved with his airway due to the mediastinal mass. I would continue to reassure him that this is the safest way. If he still doesn't allow me to perform an awake fiberoptic, I would place all of my difficult airway equipment on standby and perform an inhalational induction with sevoflurane while maintaining spontaneous ventilation.

4. **After securing the ETT, you suddenly lose the $EtCO_2$ tracing. How do you respond?**
   I would immediately manually ventilate the patient to assess the compliance of the airway as well as provide positive pressure breaths with 100% oxygen. If I still couldn't ventilate or I suspected mass compression as the etiology, I would attempt to pass a rigid bronchoscope beyond the obstruction and move the patient into the lateral or prone position to relieve the compression on the airway. Finally, if none of these maneuvers were successful, I would ask the surgeon to open the chest and begin cardiopulmonary bypass.

Hypotension

5. **Your $EtCO_2$ returns and you are able to ventilate. The procedure begins uneventfully but 15 minutes into the case, the right arterial tracing is diminished during mediastinoscopy. What do you do?**
   This is usually due to compression of the innominate artery causing artificially low BP readings. I would check a radial or femoral pulse to rule out significant

hypotension. I would also pay attention to the capnogram to rule out ventilation issues and EKG to identify any dysrhythmias that may have occurred. Assuming that the flattening of the arterial tracing is due to the innominate artery compression, I would ask the surgeon to remove the mediastinoscope while palpating for a pulse in the left arm. If those measures failed, I would begin resuscitation with fluids, blood, and pressors to restore hemodynamics.

6. **What is the relevance of facial and upper extremity edema during mediastinoscopy?**

Compression of the great vessels by a tumor in the anterior mediastinum can lead to superior vena cava syndrome. This may reduce preload with severely decreased CO. Therefore, I would ensure adequate preload prior to induction, large bore IV access in the lower extremities, and arterial line placement in the right radial artery to diagnose innominate artery compression. Because of the compromised cardiac output, avoidance of positive pressure ventilation is also warranted.

Hypoxia

7. **Thirty minutes into the procedure, you lose your pulse oximeter reading. How do you respond? What is your differential?**

I would immediately look at my other vital signs and make sure the patient is not hypotensive or hypocarbic, and has not developed any arrhythmias. I would also listen for bilateral breath sounds to rule out pneumothorax, which is a recognized complication of mediastinoscopy. I would also take the patient off the ventilator and manually ventilate the patient to assess lung compliance. Concomitant loss of $EtCO_2$ would argue strongly for an airway obstruction, most likely due to mass compression on the airway. If that did not work, I would push my ETT and/or the rigid bronchoscope distal to the lesion in an attempt to relieve the compression. I would also lighten my anesthesia and awaken the patient. Ultimately, the patient may have to be turned lateral or prone to relieve the airway mass compression. If my arterial pressure also disappeared this would most likely be innominate artery compression.

Postoperative

Extubation

1. **The surgeon wants a deep extubation in an effort to evaluate vocal cord function. How do you respond?**

My preference is to extubate the patient fully awake and assess vocal cord function postoperatively. My primary concern is to avoid loss of the airway.

2. **After neuromuscular block reversal, the patient manifests weakness and respiratory distress following extubation. What are the possible causes?**
The patient could be experiencing hypoxia, hypercarbia, hypotension, or malignant arrhythmia. In addition, assuming this patient has MG as evidenced by the chronic pyridostigmine use, I would have to distinguish between a myasthenic and a cholinergic crisis. Administration of edrophonium would improve the weakness, confirming a myasthenic crisis; exacerbation of the weakness would confirm a cholinergic crisis, and reintubation may be indicated. Other causes may be inadequate reversal of neuromuscular blockers, residual anesthetics, PTX, PE, atelectasis, and pulmonary edema.

PACU

3. **The patient develops postoperative hoarseness in the PACU. How would you evaluate?**
I would immediately go to the bedside and rule out hypoxia, hypotension, hypocarbia, or malignant arrhythmia. My most immediate concern would be recurrent laryngeal nerve injury (a recognized complication of mediastinoscopy), laryngeal edema, tracheomalacia, residual neuromuscular paralysis, or myasthenic weakness. I would check my twitches to assess muscle strength, go over my anesthetic record to see what doses of narcotics and anesthetics were given, and assess whether they have worn off. Nerve injury would be a diagnosis of exclusion. Depending on the vital signs and clinical picture, I would provide supplemental oxygen and have my intubating equipment on standby.

4. **The patient developed a left-sided hemiparesis following the procedure. The surgeon asks if this could be a myasthenic crisis. How do you respond?**
I would inform the surgeon that this is most likely not a myasthenic crisis because postoperative weakness from myasthenia gravis usually is global in nature. This focal deficit strongly points to a right-sided cerebrovascular event, most likely caused by intraoperative hypotension, air/hemorrhagic embolism, or cerebral ischemia from right innominate artery compression.

FURTHER READING

Gothard J. W. W. Anesthetic considerations for patients with anterior mediastinal masses. *Anesthesiol Clin* 2008; 26: 305–314.

Slinger P., Karsil C. Management of patients with a large anterior mediastinal mass: recurring myths. *Curr Opin Anesthesiol* 2007; 20: 1–3.

Aortic dissection

Ruchir Gupta

STEM 1

A 55 year old male is brought to the OR for emergent repair of a thoracic aortic dissection.

HPI: Patient is an actor who during his rehearsal complained of a nonspecific ripping chest pain that radiated to the neck.

PMH: Hypertension, hypercholesterolemia.

Meds: Enalapril, Lipitor.

Allergies: NKDA.

PE: VS – BP 175/85 mmHg, HR 120 bpm, RR 18, O_2 saturation 98% on 2 L/min O_2, T 37°C.

Airway – Mallampati III, thyromental distance <6 cm.

CV – tachycardic, 2/6 diastolic murmur.

CXR: Widened mediastinum.

Labs: Hct 31%; coagulation profile is normal.

Rapid Review Anesthesiology Oral Boards, ed. Ruchir Gupta and Minh Chau Joseph Tran. Published by Cambridge University Press. © Cambridge University Press 2013.

Preoperative

Heart murmur

1. **What do you think is the cause of the diastolic murmur in this patient?**
   Based on the information given it is difficult to conclude definitively about the cause of the murmur. If this is a new onset murmur, then quite possibly the aortic dissection may be extending into the aortic valve and causing aortic regurgitation. However, if this diastolic murmur were present even before this event, then it could be from mitral or tricuspid stenosis.

Classification for dissection

2. **Describe the Debakey classification system for aortic dissection.**
   The Debakey classification is as follows:
   Type I – begins in the ascending aorta and extends to the abdominal aorta.
   Type II – begins and remains in the ascending aorta.
   Type III – originates beyond the left subclavian artery and extends to the diaphragm (IIIA) or the aortoiliac bifurcation (IIIB).
   Types I and II are considered surgical emergencies whereas type III is a medical emergency.

Preoperative

3. **What further information regarding this patient's preoperative history would you want to know?**
   I would want to know more about this patient's cardiac, pulmonary, and renal status. For the cardiac, I would want to know whether this patient has had any recent stress tests or echocardiograms, recent episodes of chest pain or dyspnea at rest, and whether his murmur is new or chronic. For the pulmonary, I would want to know if this patient is a smoker or has any signs or symptoms of COPD because this patient will most likely remain intubated postoperatively. Finally, the presence of renal dysfunction is the single most important predictor of the development of renal failure after surgery. Thus, I would want a baseline BUN/creatinine in this patient.

4. **If time permitted, would you want PFTs in this patient?**
   No. The patient's respiratory status can be assessed with a thorough history and physical and I do not believe PFTs would give me any additional information that would affect my acute management.

OR setup

5. **What instructions would you give your first year anesthesia resident regarding OR room setup for this case?**

This is a case with a potential for massive blood loss and hemodynamic fluctuations. Thus, I would tell my resident to have the following items set up in the room: at least 4 NS spiked IVs, 4 units of PRBCs typed and crossed in the room with another 4 units on hold from the blood bank, a central line, TEE, arterial line, rapid transfuser, cell saver, and a crash cart in the event defibrillation/cardioversion becomes necessary. I would also ask the resident to have nitroglycerin and norepinephrine drips set up in anticipation of the aortic cross-clamp.

Intraoperative

Monitoring

1. **How would you monitor this patient?**

In addition to the standard ASA monitors, I would place a central line for volume resuscitation and CVP monitoring, a TEE to assess cardiac function, an arterial line for continuous BP monitoring as well as frequent ABGs, and a Foley catheter.

2. **Assuming you decide to place an arterial line, where would you place it?**

I would not place one, but instead two arterial lines so that I can assess the BP proximal and distal to the clamp. The proximal a-line would be placed in the right radial artery because the left subclavian artery may be clamped during the surgery, impairing blood flow to the left arm. The distal a-line could be placed in either femoral artery.

Airway

3. **How will you secure this patient's airway?**

Since the patient seems like a difficult airway, I would perform an awake fiberoptic intubation with airway nerve blocks and adequate airway topicalization with 4% nebulized lidocaine. I will have a nitroglycerin drip on standby to prevent sudden blood pressure swings during the procedure.

4. **You decide to perform an awake fiberoptic intubation (AFOI) but as you are about to begin, the surgeon yells that there is no time for an AFOI. How would you respond?**

I would inform the surgeon that there is no faster technique for securing the airway that is also safe for a patient with a suspected difficult airway. Failure to secure the airway can result in apnea, hypoxia, and death. Thus, although this may be an emergency, it is important to do what is safe for the patient.

5. **You successfully intubate the patient. Thirty minutes later, the surgeon informs you that he will be placing the cross-clamp on the aorta in the next few minutes. What hemodynamic fluctuations should you prepare for?**

The hemodynamic changes I would expect are as follows:

Proximal to the clamp: increased afterload, increased BP to upper half of body, increased CVP and pulmonary artery occlusion pressure, and decreased CO and EF.

Distal to the clamp: decreased RBF and mesenteric blood flow.

Overall there would be increased mixed venous oxygenation, decreased O_2 consumption, metabolic acidosis, and increased catecholamine release.

Aortic cross-clamp

6. **As soon as the surgeon places the cross-clamp, the BP rises to 210/110 mmHg. What are you going to do?**

The desire to treat the abrupt increase in BP, which is most likely due to an acute increase in afterload, must be weighed against the risk of reducing perfusion pressure distal to the cross-clamp. Thus I would attempt to gently reduce the afterload with an infusion of nitroglycerin or sodium nitroprusside while paying close attention to the perfusion pressure distal to the cross-clamp.

7. **Your resident begins a nitroglycerin infusion but the patient begins to develop tachycardia. What will you do?**

I will have my resident stop the infusion because tachycardia is a known side effect of nitroglycerin. Instead, I will switch to an esmolol drip to lower the BP and the HR.

8. **As you lower the BP, your arterial line in the lower extremity gives you a reading of 75/45 mmHg while the proximal arterial line reading is still elevated. What would you do?**

After confirming that both readings were accurate, I would attempt to improve the perfusion pressure distal to the cross-clamp by asking the surgeon to place a shunt, reimplant arteries to perfuse vital organs such as the kidney, spinal cord and liver, and institute hypothermia.

My target would be to try to maintain a MAP of 100 mmHg proximal to the clamp and 50 mmHg distal to the clamp.

9. **You are able to maintain stable hemodynamics during the cross-clamp portion of the surgery. The surgeon immediately removes the cross-clamp without telling you and the BP plummets to 70/40 mmHg. ST changes are noted on the EKG. What are you going to do?**

I would instruct the surgeon to immediately reapply the clamp. Once the BP improves, I will ask him to slowly and incrementally remove the clamp while I begin an infusion of norepinephrine or phenylephrine to increase the patient's SVR and to tolerate the effects of unclamping.

Postoperative

Extubation

1. Will you extubate this patient?

I would not extubate this patient because he has undergone a major vascular operation with likely blood loss and massive fluid shifts. Additionally, the incision wound is quite painful and may impair his ventilation. Thus, the risks of extubation outweigh the benefits in this case. I would leave the patient intubated overnight and gradually wean him once his fluid shifts have stabilized.

Hypothermia

2. Upon arrival in the PACU, the temperature is only 35°C. What are the immediate effects of hypothermia?

Hypothermia causes a number of deleterious effects including hyperglycemia due to a decrease in plasma insulin, decreased volume due to cold-induced diuresis, decreased platelet functions, and decreased drug metabolism.

3. How would you treat this patient's hypothermia?

I would place a Bair Hugger on the patient and administer fluids through a fluid warmer. I would also place some heated blankets around his head and consider calling to have the PACU itself warmed.

Delayed awakening

4. You turn off all sedatives in an effort to awaken the patient over the course of the next several hours. However, the patient remains unresponsive. What will you do?

Delayed awakening in this patient can be a very ominous sign because the hemodynamic fluctuations could have resulted in ischemia to the brain and spinal cord. I would initially evaluate the patient to ensure he is not hypoxic, hypotensive, or in a malignant rhythm. After that, I would review the anesthesia chart as well as the nurse's notes to see what medicines were given, including pain medicine, that can still be lingering. I would check my twitches to make sure the patient is adequately reversed. I will also send off labs including an ABG and electrolytes to make sure the patient is not hypoglycemic or anemic. Finally, if all of this is negative, I will send the patient for an emergent CT scan of the head.

FURTHER READING

Ghansah J. N., Murphy J. T. Complications of major aortic and lower extremity vascular surgery. *Semin Cardiothorac Vasc Anesth* 2004; 8(4): 335–361.

Shine T. S., Murray M. J. Intraoperative management of aortic aneurysm surgery. *Anesthesiol Clin North Am* 2004; 22(2): 289–305.

Yao F. F., Artusio, J. F. (eds.). *Yao and Artusio's Anesthesiology, Problem-Oriented Patient Management*, 6th edn. Philadelphia, PA: Lippincott Williams & Wilkins, 2008.

28

Carotid endarterectomy

Ruchir Gupta and Jaspreet Singh Toor

STEM 2

A 66 year old, 70 kg male is scheduled for a left carotid endarterectomy. He has a history of coronary artery disease, hypertension, and hypercholesterolemia. His BP is 126/80 mmHg, pulse 74 bpm, RR 15, SaO_2 96% on RA. He is currently on metoprolol, Lipitor, and HCTZ.

Preoperative

Cardiac

1. **How would you evaluate this patient's cardiac status?**
   First, I would perform a history and physical. From the history, I would want to know what this patient's baseline exercise tolerance is, as evidenced by how many flights of stairs he can climb before becoming short of breath. I would also ask him if he has any chest pain at rest. From the physical, I would want to know if there is evidence of fluid overload such as JVD or pedal edema, which would strongly suggest congestive heart failure. I would also look at a recent EKG and compare it to an old one if available, and also look for the results of any echocardiogram and stress tests he may have had. I would also speak with his cardiologist, if available.

Rapid Review Anesthesiology Oral Boards, ed. Ruchir Gupta and Minh Chau Joseph Tran. Published by Cambridge University Press. © Cambridge University Press 2013.

Hypertension

2. **How does this patient's history of hypertension affect your anesthetic management?**

Hypertension is a multisystemic disease and therefore it is important to know what organ systems are affected in this patient and then adjust my anesthetic plan accordingly.

Neuro – hypertension shifts the cerebral autoregulatory curve to the right, so what would normally be acceptable at the lower range of MAP may not be applicable in this patient. Thus, I would avoid lowering the BP to more than 20% from baseline.

Cardiac – prolonged untreated hypertension can lead to left ventricular hypertrophy and increased myocardial workload. I would review my EKG to see if there was evidence of LVH.

Renal – hypertension can be a cause of renal failure, thus if there was evidence of renal compromise, I would avoid drugs which are renally excreted and check the K^+ level.

3. **What if the patient came to the OR with a BP of 160/90 mmHg?**

I would compare it to the patient's baseline and if the BP is acutely elevated, I would probe for the cause. If this were chronic, I would hesitate to lower it because in the event that this patient has critical carotid stenosis, an elevated BP may be necessary to maintain cerebral perfusion. If this were acute, I would determine what the cause was; if anxiety, I would give midazolam, if pain, I would consider a pain reliever. I would also obtain a 12-lead EKG to rule out any myocardial events.

4. **What if the BP is 210/120 mmHg?**

I would obviously be more concerned as this is a hypertensive emergency, which is defined as a diastolic blood pressure greater than or equal to 120 mmHg and/or systolic blood pressure greater than or equal to 180 mmHg. Though I would apply the same principles as I mentioned in my previous response, I would be more aggressive in lowering this patient's BP with labetalol or even nitroglycerin.

5. **Are you concerned that lowering the BP from 210/120 mmHg may compromise cerebral perfusion?**

It is unlikely that such an elevated BP is absolutely necessary to maintain cerebral perfusion. Though I would discuss with the surgeon the extent of this patient's carotid stenosis, I would certainly want to lower the BP somewhat because at this level the patient runs the risk of a hemorrhagic stroke. Additionally, given this patient's history of CAD, the increased afterload on the heart as a result of this BP will increase the workload on the heart and increase this patient's risk of a myocardial infarction.

Neurologic

6. **Would you perform a neurologic evaluation on this patient?**
   Yes I would. Because this patient has a history of carotid stenosis, I would be interested to know if this patient has had any TIAs or symptoms of stroke. If so, I would want to know if there is any muscle weakness or any other neurologic sequelae from these incidents.

7. **Let's suppose the patient had right arm weakness from a stroke he suffered 2 years ago. How would that affect your anesthetic care?**
   If this patient had a stroke with a right arm weakness, I would avoid using that extremity for monitors such as a BP cuff or a twitch monitor and placement of IV lines. In addition, I would avoid giving this patient succinylcholine because I am worried about denervation sensitivity from the stroke causing life-threatening hyperkalemia in this patient.

Intraoperative

Anesthesia

1. **Would you perform a regional or a general anesthetic for this case?**
   There is no clear preferred method. The main benefit of regional anesthesia is that it provides us with an awake patient, which allows us to better monitor the cerebral as well as cardiac status of the patient. Additionally, hemodynamic instability associated with induction and maintenance of general anesthesia is avoided. The disadvantages of regional are the potential need for emergency intubation during the case, complications related to the cervical block, and possible patient movement during the case. The patient's anxiety level must also be assessed prior to administering regional anesthesia because extremely anxious patients may not be able to remain still for the duration of the case.

2. **If you did decide to do regional anesthesia, which block would you do?**
   A superficial and deep cervical block.

3. **What are you going to tell the patient are possible complications related to the block?**
   I would tell the patient that there is a risk of nerve injury, a risk of bleeding by accidental puncture of a blood vessel, a risk of intravascular injection, a risk that the needle may enter the epidural space and cause a high regional, and a risk that other nerves can be blocked causing a Horner's syndrome or hemiparalysis of the diaphragm. All of these would be in addition to the risk of the nerves not being properly blocked and therefore a general anesthetic will be necessary.

Monitors

4. **What kind of monitoring are you going to employ in this patient?**
   In addition to the standard ASA monitors (pulse oximeter, NIBP, EKG, EtCO$_2$, and temperature), I would like to have an arterial line to closely and more accurately monitor his BP. If I'm doing this under general anesthesia, I would want an EEG monitor if a trained person is available to interpret the EEG tracings.

5. **What other tools could you use to monitor the patient's cerebral function?**
   Though there is no gold standard for monitoring cerebral function, an awake patient is generally the best guide. In the event that a general technique was used, several monitors exist: EEG, processed EEG, SSEP, transcranial Doppler, cerebral oximetry, jugular venous oxygen saturation, and stump pressures. However, none of them have been consistently shown to improve outcome.

6. **If the patient had a 90% occlusion of his carotid on the surgical side and a 100% occlusion on the other side, which side would you start the central line on if you had to?**
   If I had to start a central line in this situation, I would prefer to do it on the side with the 100% occlusion because if I hit the carotid artery there is no risk of further injury because the vessel is already blocked. Conversely, if I started it on the surgical side and I accidentally punctured the artery, I run the risk of total occlusion of the circulation to the brain, which would be catastrophic in this patient.

Induction

7. **How would you induce this patient if you were to use a general technique?**
   My goal in inducing this patient would be to maintain hemodynamic stability in order to avoid myocardial ischemia and maintain adequate cerebral perfusion. Thus assuming the patient has a normal airway, I would use fentanyl, lidocaine, and etomidate. After ensuring I can ventilate, I would give rocuronium for muscle relaxation, and then I would intubate.

8. **Immediately after induction, the BP suddenly plummets to 70/40 mmHg. What are you going to do?**
   I would immediately look at my EKG to make sure this wasn't a malignant rhythm. I would also check the patient's oxygenation and recycle the BP to make sure this was an accurate reading. Assuming all of these parameters were normal, I would open my fluids and give a low dose vasopressor such as phenylephrine to improve the BP.

Cerebral ischemia

9. **What is meant by watershed areas?**

   Watershed areas are those areas of the circulation that lie on the border between the two carotid arteries. Their significance is that during carotid cross-clamp, it is hoped that perfusion from the non-clamped carotid artery will be sufficient to prevent a stroke in the patient. However, if the patient has poor perfusion from the non-clamped carotid artery, then there is a high likelihood of a stroke in the "watershed" areas.

10. **During the placement of the cross-clamp, the EEG technician tells you that there are changes in the EEG waveform. How do you respond?**

    I would look at my monitors and make sure the patient is not hypoxic, hyper- or hypocarbic, or hypotensive. I would also look at my inhalation agents to make sure the MAC value is less than 0.5. I would then inform the surgeon of these changes and assess if the patient is bleeding profusely as anemia can also cause such changes. If all of these things were negative, then I would ask the surgeon to release the cross-clamp.

11. **The surgeon states he cannot release the cross-clamp at such a crucial part of the procedure. How do you respond?**

    I would ask him to then place a shunt to allow some blood flow to reach the brain from the carotid artery.

12. **Why not place a shunt prophylactically in all patients undergoing this surgery?**

    Placement of these shunts is not without risks. They can serve as conduits for the movement of small thromboemboli into the neuro circulation and result in life-threatening strokes.

Postoperative

Postoperative airway distress

1. **You are paged to the PACU because the nurse says she is noticing a swelling near the surgical site. What are you going to do?**

   I would immediately go the patient's bedside and evaluate the patient. I would look at the vitals to make sure they are stable, evaluate the airway to insure that there is no airway compromise, make sure the patient is not complaining of stridor or difficulty swallowing, and examine the site of the swelling to see if it is contained or expanding. While notifying the surgeon, I would delineate the margins of the swelling with a marking pen so that I could assess whether the swelling was expanding. If time permitted, I would also send for a CBC and a coagulation profile.

2. **The patient develops stridor and complains that he is having some difficulty breathing. How would you respond?**

   I would immediately place the patient on 100% oxygen via face mask and prepare to emergently intubate the patient at the bedside while calling for help and the difficult airway cart. I would also look at the surgical site to see if it has continued to expand and have the surgeon paged emergently so we could evacuate any hematoma.

3. **Besides a hematoma, what are the other causes of stridor in a post-endarterectomy patient?**

   Besides external compression from a hematoma, it could also be from residual anesthetics like inadequate reversal of muscle relaxants and inhalation agents as well as an overdose of postoperative opioid administration.

Postoperative hypertension

4. **During a routine postoperative visit, you notice the BP is 190/100 mmHg. How will you respond?**

   A malfunctioning carotid sinus is common after these procedures. I would immediately go to the bedside and confirm that this is an accurate reading while assessing the other vital signs to rule out hypoxia, hypercarbia, or a malignant rhythm including MI. Next, assuming these were normal, I would try to assess the cause: is the patient anxious or in any discomfort? If no clear etiology could be determined, I would infuse a beta blocker such as labetalol.

5. **The surgeon asks if the patient needs to be transferred to the ICU or whether he can be transferred to the general medical floor. How do you respond?**

   I would want this patient to be transferred to the ICU because this patient is at high risk for hemodynamic instability from the endarterectomy. In addition, given the recent episode of a hematoma in the neck, I would want to watch this patient closely to assure there is no reaccumulation of blood and that the patient does not develop any more episodes of stridor.

FURTHER READING

Atchabahian A., Gupta R. (eds.). *The Anesthesia Guide*. New York: McGraw-Hill Publishing, 2013.

Barash P. G., Cullen B. F., Stoelting R. K., Cahalan M., Stock, C. M. (eds.). *Clinical Anesthesia*, 6th edn. Philadelphia, PA: Lippincott Williams & Wilkins, 2009.

Ho M. D. *The Essential Oral Board Review*, 3rd edn. Houston, TX: Anesthesiology Consultants, 2003.

Thiesen G. J. Grundy B. L. Anesthesia and monitoring for carotid endarterectomy. *Bull NY Acad Med* 1987; 63(8): 803–819.

29

Coronary artery bypass graft (CABG)

Ruchir Gupta

STEM 1

A 69 year old, 70 kg male presents to the operating room for a four-vessel coronary artery bypass graft (CABG).

HPI: The patient has thus far been asymptomatic but had a positive stress test during a routine check-up. Cardiac catheterization revealed severe four-vessel disease with >80% occlusion. His echocardiogram revealed an ejection fraction (EF) of 40%.

PMH: Type 2 diabetes mellitus; hypertension; hypercholesterolemia.

Meds: Metoprolol, nitroglycerin infusion, metformin, Lipitor.

Allergies: Penicillin.

PE: Vital signs – P 85 bpm, BP 110/67 mmHg, RR 14, O_2 saturation 96% on RA.

Airway – Mallampati II, full cervical ROM, teeth intact.

Lungs – clear to auscultation bilaterally.

CV – regular rate, no murmurs.

EKG: Multiple Q waves in inferolateral leads, ST depression in V4–V6.

CXR: Normal, no active infiltrates/effusions.

Labs: Hb 12 g/dL, Plt 250k, glucose 120 mg/dL.

Rapid Review Anesthesiology Oral Boards, ed. Ruchir Gupta and Minh Chau Joseph Tran. Published by Cambridge University Press. © Cambridge University Press 2013.

Preoperative

Myocardial ischemia

1. **Based on the information given, does it seem possible that this patient could have suffered from silent heart attacks in the past?**
   Yes, the appearance of Q waves strongly suggests prior heart attacks. In addition, patients with diabetes often develop silent MIs secondary to diabetic induced neuropathies which damage myocardial pain fibers. Finally, this patient has several risk factors for an MI including HTN, hypercholesterolemia, and DM. Thus, most likely this patient has had silent MIs in the past.

2. **How does a patient develop myocardial ischemia?**
   Myocardial ischemia develops whenever there is an imbalance between supply and demand of oxygenated blood to the myocardium. In CAD, patients often have coronary plaques that result in luminal narrowing of the arteries. With time, shearing forces from blood flow against the plaques result in clot formation with resultant total occlusion of the coronary artery. Heart muscle suffers from ischemia with possible progression to infarction as a result.

Beta blockers

3. **Describe the ACC/AHA recommendations for perioperative beta blockers.**
   The ACC/AHA recommendations are that beta blockers should be continued in patients already receiving beta blockers who undergo intermediate risk or vascular surgery and have a history of CAD, or high cardiac risk as defined by ischemic heart disease, DM, cerebrovascular disease, or CHF.

Diabetes

4. **A hemoglobin A1C (HbA1C) level comes at 8.4%. How does this information affect your anesthetic management?**
   This level is extremely high and indicates that the patient has poorly controlled diabetes. I would be concerned about complications arising from poorly controlled diabetes; for example, atlanto-occipital joint stiffness can make intubation challenging, renal insufficiency from diabetic nephropathy may necessitate the use of drugs that do not undergo renal clearance, widespread peripheral vascular disease may predispose this patient to a stroke and diabetic ulcers, and gastroparesis would make him a full stomach.

Preoperative sedation

5. **Would you give this patient any sedatives preoperatively?**
   It depends on the anxiety level of the patient. If I feel the patient is relatively comfortable and relaxed, I would not administer any sedatives because of the

possible risk of hypotension. However, if the patient were extremely anxious, I would worry about the effects anxiety can have on the patient's cardiac status (i.e., tachycardia, HTN) and so in that scenario the benefits would outweigh the risk of administering an anxiolytic.

Intraoperative

Monitoring

1. **What kind of monitoring will you use for this patient?**
   I will place the standard ASA monitors (including a five-lead EKG), a PAC, a CVP, a TEE, and a preinduction arterial line.

Induction

2. **Is propofol an appropriate induction agent for this patient?**
   Propofol would not be my first choice for inducing this patient. Its hypotensive properties will aggravate the severe CAD and further impair perfusion to the myocardium, resulting in a decreased supply to demand ratio in a patient with an already diseased myocardium.

3. **Etomidate is on back order. You decide to use propofol to induce this patient. Suddenly, the BP drops to 75/50 mmHg and HR rises to 110 bpm. How do you respond?**
   I would immediately look at the other vital signs and make sure the patient is not hypoxic, hypercarbic, or in a malignant arrhythmia. I will also open my fluids wide, place the patient in Trendelenburg position, and administer small doses of a vasoconstrictor such as phenylephrine to temporize.

Heparin

4. **The surgeon asks you to give heparin in preparation for the bypass. What heparin dose will you give?**
   The initial starting dose is 3–4 units/kg, but the effect of this dose varies patient to patient. Thus, after administering the standard dose, I will check the ACT level, aiming for an ACT of >300 seconds. If this has not been achieved, I will administer additional boluses of heparin.

5. **Your ACT level comes back at 130 seconds. Is this adequate? If not, what will you do?**
   No. The target ACT level in this patient is >300 seconds. Thus, I will probe for causes for such a low ACT such as incorrect drug administered, kinked/infiltrated IV tubing, erroneous ACT measurement, or possibly heparin resistance.

Bypass considerations

6.   **Your resident asks you about the benefits of on-pump CABG versus off-pump CABG (OPCAB). How do you respond?**
     I would tell my resident that the main benefit of OPCAB is the avoidance of the CPB machine with its resulting systemic effects which include the inflammatory response, neurologic injury, coagulopathies, platelet dysfunction, fibrinolysis, renal impairment, and arrhythmias such as atrial fibrillation. OPCAB has been shown to have similar graft patency and overall better results than conventional surgery in high-risk patients.
     Conversely, the benefit of on-pump CABG is that the procedure is easier to perform technically by the surgeon and hemodynamic changes can be managed by the perfusionist and the bypass machine more easily than when such changes happen in a beating heart.

7.   **At the start of bypass, you notice the patient's BP is 90/60 mmHg. What would you do?**
     I would initially make sure the patient was not hypoxic by checking the pulse oximeter. I would immediately notify the perfusionist of this low BP because hypotension during bypass is usually due to either low cardiac output or low SVR. Thus, if the CO were low, I would ask the perfusionist to increase the pump flow rate. If the issue was peripheral resistance, I would administer a vasoconstrictor such as phenylephrine.

8.   **Describe what steps you would take to wean the patient off bypass.**
     In preparation for coming off bypass, I would begin rewarming to ensure normothermia, administer midazolam to prevent awareness during rewarming, turn on my anesthesia monitors and alarms, correct any lab abnormalities such as anemia and electrolyte disturbances, ensure the heart is de-aired, initiate ventilation, check the TEE to assess cardiac function, and have a pacing device on standby.

Heparin reversal

9.   **What medicine is routinely given to reverse the effect of heparin? What dose would you use?**
     Protamine is routinely used and its dose is 1 mg/100 units of heparin.

10. **How does protamine reverse the effects of heparin?**
     Heparin is an acid and protamine is a base. Thus, they interact to form an inactive salt.

Postoperative

Ventilatory modes

1. **You take the patient to the ICU intubated. What ventilator setting would you use? Why?**

   It depends on the course of the surgery. If this was a routine CABG and there were no unforeseen events, I would place the patient on a weaning mode of ventilation, such as synchronized intermittent mandatory ventilation (SIMV). However, if this case were complicated by an intraoperative event, I might want to keep this patient sedated and on controlled ventilation.

Postoperative bleeding

2. **You notice that in the first hour since transferring the patient to the cardiac ICU, there has been over 300 mL of blood drainage through the chest tube. What do you think is occurring?**

   There can be several causes of coagulopathy in this patient: thrombocytopenia, hypothermia, dilution of coagulation factors, DIC, and inadequate heparin reversal.

3. **Your resident has a protamine syringe in his hand and is about to administer it. How do you respond?**

   I would immediately tell him to stop. In order to determine the cause of this coagulopathy, further tests need to be done including a CBC with platelets, coagulation profile, fibrinogen level with fibrin split products, and an ACT. Only after receiving all of the results can we be sure of the etiology.

4. **Your resident asks you if he could just give protamine now in case it was an issue with heparin reversal. How do you respond?**

   I would tell him that protamine is not without risks and can lead to anaphylactic/anaphylactoid reactions, pulmonary hypertension, hypotension, and even myocardial depression. Thus it should not be used as empiric therapy for a possible diagnosis. Only a definitive diagnosis, guided by an ACT, can guide therapy.

FURTHER READING

Gupta R. *Anesthesiology Pocketcard Set*. Germany: Borm Bruckmeir Publishing, 2009.

Miller R. D., Eriksson L. I., Fleisher L. A., Wiener-Kornish J. P., Young W. L. (eds.). *Miller's Anesthesia*, 7th edn. Philadelphia, PA: Churchill Livingstone Elsevier, 2010.

Virmani S., Tempe D. Anesthesia for off pump coronary artery surgery. *Ann Card Anesth* 2007; 10: 65–71.

www.netdoc.com/Medical-News/general-surgery/ACC%10AHA-release-revised-guidelines-for-beta-blockers/.

30

Abdominal aortic aneurysm

Ruchir Gupta

STEM 2

A 55 year old, 75 kg male presents to the operating room for an open repair of an abdominal aortic aneurysm. A CT of the abdomen shows the size of the aneurysm to be 7.5 cm. Patient has a 50 pack year smoking history, HTN, CAD, and COPD. His medications include albuterol, lisinopril, HCTZ, and ASA. Vital signs: BP 150/65 mmHg, HR 88 bpm, RR 18, O_2 saturation 98% on RA. Hb 12.2 g/dL.

Preoperative

Labs

1. **What other preoperative labs, if any, would you want in this patient?**
   In addition to the Hb value, I would want a coagulation profile in case a thoracic epidural were to be placed, metabolic panel to rule out any electrolyte disturbances, and a baseline ABG to assess the severity of his COPD.

Respiratory

2. **Do you need PFTs?**
   No, I would not rush to obtain PFTs because most of the information I need to know about this patient's respiratory status can be elicited from a focused history and physical.

Rapid Review Anesthesiology Oral Boards, ed. Ruchir Gupta and Minh Chau Joseph Tran. Published by Cambridge University Press. © Cambridge University Press 2013.

Cardiovascular

3. Are you going to lower this patient's blood pressure preoperatively?

An elevated BP predisposes this patient's aneurysm to rupture, so I would want to lower it but I have to balance my desire to prevent an aneurysm rupture against the risk of decreasing myocardial perfusion in a patient with heart disease. Thus, I will lower it by up to 20% from baseline and attempt to maintain the patient's BP at that level.

4. How will you evaluate this patient's cardiac status?

I will go to the bedside and perform a focused history and physical. From the history, I want to assess his METs level and baseline symptomatology. I would also inquire about previous history of myocardial infarction, interventional procedures such as cardiac stent placement, and use of anticoagulation. From the physical, I will look for signs of heart failure such as fluid overload or pulmonary edema. Finally, if available, I would like to see the results of a recent stress test or an echocardiogram.

5. Do you need an echocardiogram before taking this patient to the OR?

It depends on the results of my history and physical. If the patient has no signs of heart failure such as JVD, pedal edema, or pulmonary edema, and lives an active lifestyle and has an otherwise normal physical exam, I would forgo obtaining an echo. If, however, he displayed signs of fluid overload, had a sedentary lifestyle, and presented with an undiagnosed heart murmur on physical exam, I would want an echocardiogram if time permitted.

Beta blockers

6. Would you administer a beta blocker to this patient on the day of surgery if he has not been on one?

Yes. I would give a beta-1-selective agent such as metoprolol because of his COPD, titrated to heart rate and blood pressure for this patient with a CAD history who is about to undergo a major vascular operation.

Intraoperative

Monitoring

1. What monitors will you place on this patient?

In addition to the standard ASA monitors, I would want a preinduction a-line to monitor the BP closely, a central line for CVP monitoring and massive fluid resuscitation, a PAC to monitor cardiac filling pressures during aortic cross-clamp, and a Foley catheter. If a TEE were available, I would use it in lieu of the PAC.

2. **Your patient is extremely nervous about having any needles placed in him preoperatively. Would you assure the patient that the arterial line will be placed only after he is asleep?**

   No, I will want to place this patient's a-line prior to induction. To alleviate his anxiety, I will reassure the patient verbally, and if needed, titrate a small dose of an anxiolytic such as midazolam. I will also inject local anesthesia prior to placing the a-line.

Induction

3. **Will you use propofol for induction?**

   No. Propofol would not be my first choice because it can result in life-threatening hypotension. My goal for induction is to maintain the BP at 20% from baseline. Thus, I would rather use etomidate in this patient.

Nitroprusside toxicity

4. **As the surgeon is about to place the aortic cross-clamp, you start a nitroprusside infusion. What are some possible toxic effects of nitroprusside?**

   Nitroprusside is associated with the development of cyanomethemoglobin, thiocyanate, and cyanide toxicity which results in an impairment of oxygen utilization. As a result, the patient develops metabolic acidosis, cardiac arrhythmias, and tachyphylaxis.

5. **How is nitroprusside toxicity treated?**

   Nitroprusside toxicity is treated with supportive measures such as discontinuing the infusion, ventilation with 100% oxygen, and the administration of drugs that neutralize the nitroprusside molecules: sodium thiosulfate, inhaled amyl nitrate, and hydroxocobalamin.

Aortic cross-clamp

6. **What are some adverse effects of aortic cross-clamp?**

   Aortic cross-clamping results in a massive increase in afterload proximal to the clamp and a decrease in perfusion distal to the clamp. As a result, there is a massive strain on the myocardium with increase in cardiac filling pressure. There is also an increased risk of renal failure, bowel ischemia, and spinal cord ischemia.

7. **Your resident asks you if placing the aortic cross-clamp below the renal arteries will offer better renal protection than placing it above. How do you respond?**

   Infrarenal cross-clamping does not offer renal protection because there is an increase in renal vascular resistance. As a result, renal blood flow decreases and ischemic injuries still occur.

8. **Shortly after the release of the aortic cross-clamp, you notice the patient's blood pressure suddenly plummets to 80/45 mmHg with an HR of 45 bpm. What will you do?**

   I will immediately rule out hypoxia as the cause and look at my EKG rhythm to rule out a malignant arrhythmia. Assuming the patient has a pulse and the rhythm is sinus, I will immediately send for a transcutaneous pacer while administering atropine, epinephrine, and fluids as a temporizing measure.

Postoperative

Hypotension

1. **You take the patient to the PACU intubated and over the next hour the nurse tells you that the patient's BP has been gradually decreasing to 90/55 mmHg while the HR has gradually trended upward to 110 bpm. What will you do?**

   I will immediately go to the bedside and ensure that the patient is adequately oxygenating and ventilating. I will also look at my EKG to rule out any malignant arrhythmia. Assuming these are all normal, I will check my CVP and Foley catheter to assess the fluid status to see if this patient is hypovolemic. If so, I'll administer fluids wide open. I will send a CBC to rule out anemia and check any drains or sheets to see if the patient is bleeding. If this is the case, I will transfuse with PRBCs. I will also alert the surgeon while I am conducting my assessment in case we need to rush the patient back to the OR.

Delayed awakening

2. **The issue resolves. One hour later you are again paged to the PACU because the patient is unresponsive even though the sedation was stopped 30 minutes ago. How will you respond?**

   I will immediately go to the bedside and ensure the patient has stable vital signs and is not hypoxic, hypercarbic, hypotensive, or in a malignant arrhythmia. I will also look at the PACU nurse's notes to see what pain medicine or sedative had been used. I will check a train of four to ensure the patient has been adequately reversed and check my anesthesia record for the last time any drugs were given. Finally, I will send off a CBC to rule out anemia, a metabolic panel to rule out electrolyte disturbances including hypoglycemia, and an ABG to rule out any acid–base disturbance as an etiology. If my focused neurologic exam points towards a stroke, I will send the patient for a STAT head CT.

3. **What role could aortic cross-clamping have played in this finding?**

   Hemodynamic fluctuations caused by aortic cross-clamping could have led to a hemorrhagic or an ischemic stroke in this patient.

ABG interpretation

4. **An ABG performed a few hours later shows a pH of 7.30, PaCO$_2$ 50 mmHg, PaO$_2$ 60 mmHg, HCO$_3$ 26 mEq/L on 50% oxygen. Interpret.**
   This is an uncompensated respiratory acidosis with hypoxemia.

5. **What will you do?**
   I will immediately go to the bedside and examine the patient. First, I will check the circuit to make sure there are no kinks or occlusions, and that the ETT has not become mainstem by auscultating the lungs. Assuming all these things are normal, I will examine the patient to see if he is hypoventilating. I will recommend switching the patient to controlled ventilation mode if he is not already on it and consider increasing tidal volume and respiratory rate as tolerated. I will also repeat my ABG prior to making any changes.

FURTHER READING

Atchabahian A., Gupta R. (eds.). *The Anesthesia Guide*. New York: McGraw-Hill Publishing, 2013.
Higgens T. L. Quantifying risk and assessing outcome in cardiac surgery. *J Cardiothorac Vasc Anesth* 1998; 12: 330.

31

Hemorrhage

Edouard Belotte

STEM 1

A 32 year old G2P1 with twin gestation presents to the obstetric floor for vaginal bleeding.

HPI: Her previous pregnancy resulted in a cesarean section, but she had hoped for a vaginal delivery this time for her 36 week gestation twins.

PMH: Gestational diabetes, COPD.

SH: 10 pack year smoker, did not smoke during pregnancy.

PE: VS – P 87 bpm, RR 18, BP 120/76 mmHg, O_2 97% on RA.

Airway – Mallampati III, full cervical range of motion.

CV – regular rate and rhythm.

Pulmonary – clear to auscultation.

Labs: Hb 9.1 g/dL, platelets 240k, WBC 12.1k/mcL, Na 138 mEq/L, K 4.5 mEq/L.

Preoperative

Hemodynamics

1. **How would you assess this patient's hemodynamic status ?**
   I will go to the patient's bedside and perform a history and physical. From the history I would ask the patient if there are any complaints of light-headedness,

Rapid Review Anesthesiology Oral Boards, ed. Ruchir Gupta and Minh Chau Joseph Tran. Published by Cambridge University Press. © Cambridge University Press 2013.

nausea, positional vertigo, or syncopal episodes. From the physical exam, I would look at her vital signs, especially the blood pressure and HR to evaluate for hypotension and reflex tachycardia. I could also look for signs of hypovolemia such as capillary refill time, moisture of mucous membranes, and skin turgor to determine if this patient's blood loss has resulted in hypovolemia with progression to hemodynamic instability.

Bleeding etiology

2. What is the differential diagnosis of third trimester bleeding?
The most common causes of third trimester hemorrhage are placenta previa and placental abruption. Placenta previa is the abnormal implantation of the placenta in front of the fetal presenting part. Placental abruption is separation of the placenta from the decidua basalis before delivery of the fetus. There is a strong association between a previous uterine scar and the development of placenta previa.

Less common causes of antepartum hemorrhage are due to cervical pathology such as polyps, carcinoma, uterine rupture, vasa previa, and local genital tract lesions. Preeclampsia and intrauterine death place patients at risk for coagulopathies, which may give rise to maternal hemorrhage.

3. How do you distinguish a placenta previa from a placental abruption?
The definitive diagnosis of each is determined by ultrasound, but a focused history can often help make the distinction. A placenta previa will present with painless vaginal bleeding whereas placental abruption will present with painful bleeding.

4. What are the most common clinical manifestations of each?
Patients with placenta previa have painless bright red vaginal bleeding that rarely progresses to hypovolemic shock and DIC, and patients with placental abruption have port wine non-clotted painful bleeding that commonly progresses to hypovolemic shock and DIC.

Double setup

5. What is a double setup? When it is indicated?
A double setup is a vaginal examination performed in the operating room with the immediate capability of converting to cesarean section under general anesthesia. It is indicated whenever there is a real chance of needing to convert rapidly to GA. The entire obstetric team needs to be present (anesthesiologist, obstetrician, pediatrician, nurse, and surgical technician). The patient should have large bore intravenous access, standard monitoring, and appropriate anesthetic drugs available in the OR.

Uterine rupture

6. **Who is at risk for uterine rupture? How is uterine rupture diagnosed?**

   Uterine rupture is a potentially life-threatening condition that occurs in patients with previous uterine scars such as from a C-section. Risk factors include use of prostaglandins, uterine trauma, a tumultuous labor, midforceps delivery, breech version and extraction, inappropriate uterotonic use, uterine anomalies, placenta percreta, tumors, fetal macrosomia, and fetal malposition. The most consistent sign of uterine rupture is fetal distress. Other signs that may be present include hypotension, vaginal bleeding, abdominal pain, change in the uterine contour, changes in the uterine contraction pattern, and cessation of labor. True diagnosis is made either during manual inspection of the uterus or during a laparotomy.

Preoperative labs

7. **Do you want any additional laboratory assessments before taking this patient to the operating room?**

   Yes. I would order a coagulation profile (to determine suitability for neuraxial technique as well as an early indicator for DIC) and type and cross for 2 units of PRBC.

Intraoperative

Regional vs. general

1. **Would you perform a regional or a general anesthetic for this patient?**

   Based on the information given, this patient is currently hemodynamically stable. If her bleeding was not brisk and her overall blood loss had not been significant, I would want to perform an epidural on this patient. If, however, she displayed any signs of hypovolemia and/or she was actively hemorrhaging profusely I would want to avoid the sympathectomy caused by the epidural and instead opt to do this case under GA.

Monitoring

2. **What invasive monitors, if any, would you place?**

   I would place a radial arterial line to detect any abrupt changes in blood pressure as well as to allow access for blood sampling for serial hematocrit, ABG, and coagulation in the event the patient's condition deteriorates. I would also ensure that a Foley catheter is placed to assess adequacy of urine output. Finally, if I didn't have at least two 18 g PIVs or bigger, I would place a central line.

Transfusion

3. Would you transfuse blood to this patient prior to administering anesthesia?

Transfusion of blood products should be guided by the volume of blood loss over time and changes in hemodynamic parameters (e.g., blood pressure, maternal and fetal heart rates, peripheral perfusion, and urine output), as well as the hemoglobin level. Thus, assuming the patient was otherwise stable with reassuring FHR tracing, I would not rush to transfusion.

Induction

4. Assuming a general anesthetic technique is selected, how would you induce this patient for the C-section?

Because this patient is considered full stomach, I would premedicate with sodium citrate before induction of general anesthesia. After preoxygenation with 100% oxygen, I would perform a rapid sequence induction with cricoid pressure using fentanyl, etomidate, and succinylcholine.

Intraoperative hemorrhage

5. The patient is hemorrhaging after removal of the placenta. Her blood pressure reads 95/50 mmHg. Heart rate is 106 bpm and oxygen saturation is 96%. What is your management?

While recycling the blood pressure, I will open my fluids wide, place the patient in Trendelenburg position with head down, and administer a small dose of phenylephrine. I will concurrently communicate with the surgeon to determine if the hemorrhage is ongoing. If it is and the patient continues to be hypotensive, I would immediately begin the blood transfusion.

6. How would you assess for the amount of blood loss?

Blood loss needs to be assessed by looking at the operating field, communicating with the surgeon, counting the sponges, and checking the suction canister.

7. What is the role of cell salvage in obstetric patients?

The use of intraoperative cell salvage for peripartum hemorrhage is still controversial, although major obstetric anesthesia societies now regard it as an acceptable alternative to allogeneic transfusion. The fear is that amniotic fluid components will be administered to the patient and cause an amniotic fluid embolism. However, intraoperative cell salvage has nonetheless been shown to have an undisputed role in obstetrics in patients with high risk such as placenta previa/accreta, massive fibroids, or rare blood type or unusual antibodies. Intraoperative cell salvage can be also useful in the treatment of Jehovah's Witnesses. Cell saver may decrease the risk of bloodborne infections associated with transfusion of banked red blood cells (RBCs) and may also decrease the risk of alloimmunization. The risks of transfusion reactions and transfusion-related acute lung injury would also be reduced if autologous blood was used instead of banked blood.

8. **What invasive options are available to control peripartum hemorrhage when medical treatment is unsuccessful in controlling the bleeding?**
Several invasive options are available to control peripartum hemorrhage when medical treatments fail.

Uterine balloon tamponade: Uterine packing has long been the treatment of choice to manage peripartum hemorrhage; it is safe, quick, and easily performed by relatively inexperienced personnel, and can be performed with or without anesthesia.

Uterine arterial embolization: It has become a well-recognized alternative method of treatment in the conservative management of peripartum hemorrhage in association with local or medical treatment, or in the event of their failure. This therapeutic approach avoids morbidity associated with peripartum hysterectomy and preserves fertility. It is also a possible additional approach when arterial ligation or hysterectomy fails to control bleeding.

Surgical iliac (or uterine) artery ligation: When uterine tamponade and arterial embolization fail, a laparotomy to perform iliac artery ligation is an option to preserve the uterus. It can also be performed as a first invasive option, during C-section delivery, or when the patient is hemodynamically unstable or if embolization is not readily available.

B-Lynch suture: since its first description in 1997, the so-called B-Lynch uterine compression suture has been used successfully to control bleeding following failed conservative management.

Emergency hysterectomy may be required to control bleeding refractory to other methods and save lives.

Postoperative

Postpartum hemorrhage

1. **The patient is now in the PACU following the C-section. You are called to see this patient because of continuing hemorrhage. What is the definition of postpartum hemorrhage (PPH)?**
PPH is defined as blood loss of more than 500 mL following vaginal delivery or more than 1000 mL following cesarean delivery. A loss of these amounts within 24 hours of delivery is termed early or primary PPH, whereas such losses are termed late or secondary PPH if they occur 24 hours after delivery. Another proposal suggests using a 10% fall in hematocrit value to define PPH. Patients with unexplained hypotension, tachycardia, or low urine output should be suspected of having a postpartum hemorrhage, and resuscitation should commence.

2. **What is the differential diagnosis of PPH?**

PPH has many potential causes, but the most common is uterine atony (failure of the uterus to contract and retract following delivery of the baby). Other risk factors are high birthweight, labor induction and augmentation, chorioamnionitis, magnesium sulfate use, previous PPH, uterine causes such as retained products of conception, placental accreta, uterine inversion, and uterine rupture, and nonuterine causes such as genital tract lesions, genital tract hematomas, intra-abdominal lacerations, pelvic lacerations, and coagulopathies including DIC.

3. **How will you assess this patient with PPH?**

I will immediately go to the bedside and perform a focused history and physical. From the history, I would review the chart to see how much blood loss has occurred intraoperatively and postoperatively. I would also look for what fluids, pressors, and blood products she has received during this time. I would also ask the patient if she feels light-headed or nauseous and whether there is any change in her mentation. I would also look at how much urine output she has had. From the physical, I would first look at her vital signs to evaluate for hypotension and tachycardia. I would also see if she is still bleeding and look for any bloody sheets or towels. Finally, I would look for any signs of DIC (widespread bruising or hemorrhage) and order a STAT CBC, coagulation profile, d-dimer, and inform the surgeon.

FURTHER READING

Blomberg M. Maternal obesity and risk of postpartum hemorrhage. *Obstet Gynecol* 2011; 118(3): 561–568.

Clark S. L., Koonings P. P., Phelan J. P. Placenta previa/accreta and prior cesarean section. *Obstet Gynecol* 1985; 66(1): 89–92.

Gabbe S. G., Niebyl J. R., Galan H. L., Jauniaux E. R., Landon M. B., et al. *Gabbe: Obstetrics: Normal and Problem Pregnancies*, 6th edn. Philadelphia: PA. Elsevier Saunders, 2012.

Jackson K. W. Jr, Allbert J. R., Schemmer G. K., Elliot M., Humphrey A., Taylor J. A randomized controlled trial comparing oxytocin administration before and after placental delivery in the prevention of postpartum hemorrhage. *Am J Obstet Gynecol* 2001; 185(4): 873–877.

Mayer D. C., Spielman F. J., Bell E. A. Antepartum and postpartum hemorrhage. In: Chestnut D. H. (ed.), *Obstetric Anesthesia: Principles and Practice*, 3rd edn. Philadelphia, PA: Elsevier Mosby, 2004; 668–671.

Wali A., Suresh M. S., Gregg A. R. Antepartum hemorrhage. In: Datta S. (ed.), *Anesthetic and Obstetric Management of High-Risk Pregnancy*, 3rd edn. New York: Springer, 2004; 94–98.

32

Preeclampsia

Xiaodong Bao

STEM 2

A 23 year old, 85 kg, G3P1 female who is 36 weeks pregnant is admitted to the labor and delivery suite for an urgent cesarean section due to premature rupture of membrane. She has had very limited prenatal care and is not on any regular medications. Her past medical history is significant for chronic IVDA. On admission, her vital signs are: BP 150/110 mmHg, HR 100 bpm, SaO$_2$ 96% on RA. Hb 10.1 g/dL.

Preoperative

Drug abuse

1. **What are your anesthetic concerns?**
   I have concerns for both mother and fetus. Regarding the mother, I am concerned about her IVDA status. She could have poor IV access, multiple drug abuse, increase risk of transmitted diseases such as hepatitis and HIV, drug dependence and withdrawal syndrome, and systemic derangement depending on abused drugs. I am also worried about her poor prenatal care that predisposes both mother and fetus to much higher peripartum complications. She may have undiagnosed preeclampsia as evidenced by her high blood pressure. Uncontrolled hypertension and cocaine abuse substantially increases the risk of placental abruption. There is also increased chance of postpartum hemorrhage. For the fetus, I am concerned that the baby may suffer IUGR, intraventricular hemorrhage, congenital abnormalities, and low birthweight. The fetus could have sustained exposure to different abusive medications resulting in fetal dependence and withdrawal syndrome.

Rapid Review Anesthesiology Oral Boards, ed. Ruchir Gupta and Minh Chau Joseph Tran. Published by Cambridge University Press. © Cambridge University Press 2013.

2. **What are your differential diagnoses for hypertension in this patient?**

There are abundant reasons for why this patient is hypertensive. The patient may have untreated chronic hypertension, gestational hypertension, or preeclampsia, or the hypertension may be drug induced such as from cocaine or amphetamine.

3. **The patient adamantly denies any medical problems before pregnancy. She reluctantly admits that she does use cocaine frequently. Do you think the patient's elevated blood pressure is due to the cocaine abuse? How would you differentiate that from baseline preeclampsia?**

Cocaine abuse can certainly lead to sympathetic activation with maternal hypertension, tachycardia, arrhythmia, and myocardial ischemia. In fact, in severe cases, hyperreflexia and convulsions due to cocaine abuse can mimic preeclampsia/eclampsia. I would obtain a more detailed history and physical information, including routes of administration, last time of abuse, amount taken, duration of abuse, and medical treatments she has undergone. I will also look for signs of cocaine abuse use such as dilated pupils, increased heart rate, arrhythmia, and agitation. I will send out a toxicology screen as well as urine study to help me differentiate.

4. **Urine test comes back negative for cocaine. What does that mean?**

It means that the patient probably has not abused cocaine within 3–5 days.

Preeclampsia

5. **What is preeclampsia? How is that distinguished from severe preeclampsia?**

Preeclampsia is a multi-organ disorder that presents after 20 weeks gestation with remission usually by 48 hours after delivery. It is characterized by sustained SBP of at least 140 mmHg or DBP of at least 90 mmHg (more than twice, 4 to 6 hours apart) and proteinuria with 300 mg or more protein in 24 hour urine collection.

Severe preeclampsia is diagnosed if there is preeclampsia plus one of the following:

- Sustained SBP ≥160 mmHg or DBP ≥110 mmHg.
- Evidence of end organ damage.
- Deteriorating renal function including severe proteinuria (more than 5 g/24 h), sudden oliguria, especially with elevated creatinine.
- CNS disturbance (headache, vision disturbance).
- Liver dysfunction.
- Thrombocytopenia.
- HELLP.
- Epigastric/right upper quadrant pain (stretching of hepatic capsule).
- Pulmonary edema.
- Fetal compromise (IUGR, oligohydramnios, nonreassuring fetal testing).

6. **You suspect that the patient has preeclampsia. What laboratory test(s) would you like to order?**
   I will send out a CBC, BMP, liver function test to assess for HELLP syndrome, uric acid, UA, 24 hour urine protein, and a coagulation study.

Intraoperative

Magnesium therapy

1. **Should you stop the magnesium infusion prior to the procedure?**
   No. Magnesium sulfate is the first-line drug treatment for seizure prophylaxis.

2. **What are the pharmacodynamic effects of MgSO$_4$?**
   Magnesium sulfate decreases the release of acetylcholine and decreases the sensitivity of the motor end plate to acetylcholine. It has the following effects:
   - **V** – vasodilation–hypotension.
   - **A** – anticonvulsant.
   - **S** – sedative, skeletal muscle relaxant; increased sensitivity to both depolarizing and nondepolarizing muscle relaxants. Fasciculation may not be observed after succinylcholine.
   - **T** – tocolytic (decreases uterine activity) which increases uterine blood flow.

3. **What are the side effects of magnesium sulfate?**
   - Diminished deep tendon reflexes (4–5 mEq/L).
   - EKG changes including prolonged PR and ST intervals, widened QRS complexes, and/or elevated T waves (4–7 mEq/L).
   - Somnolence (5–7 mEq/L).
   - Loss of deep tendon reflexes, or myotonia (8–10 mEq/L).
   - Heart block (12 mEq/L).
   - Respiratory arrest (15 mEq/L).
   - Cardiac arrest and cardiovascular collapse (20 mEq/L).

Thrombocytopenia

4. **The platelet number comes back at 90k. Are you comfortable with placing an epidural for this case?**
   Yes, as long as this is a steady-state platelet count and there was no recent abrupt decline. A common practice has been that if platelet count is >75k, in the absence of other coagulation abnormalities, I would not expect to see an increase in neuraxial anesthetic complications in the setting of preeclampsia.

5. **If there were no previous labs studies on this patient, would you still proceed with an epidural technique with a platelet number of 75k?**
   Although I will be more alarmed at this level, I will still proceed with an epidural technique as long as the patient does not demonstrate increased bleeding

tendencies on history and physical exam. The obstetricians and patient will be counseled on the risks and benefits of the procedure prior to obtaining consent from the patient. Blood products including platelets will be in the room prior to surgical incision.

Deceleration

6. **Before performing the epidural, there is an episode of late deceleration on the FHR monitor, and the obstetric physician decides on a STAT cesarean section. How would this change your anesthetic plan?**

   I will perform a single-shot spinal for the STAT cesarean section. Traditionally, spinal anesthesia has been dreaded for inducing dramatic swings of blood pressure in preeclamptic patients. More recent studies demonstrate that single-shot spinal, combined spinal-epidural, and epidural anesthesia can all be used effectively for this patient population. In some studies, because of vasoconstriction, incidence and severity of hypotension after single-shot spinal are less in women with preeclampsia than in healthy women. In this patient, I would perform a spinal anesthetic because it provides a more dense surgical block and we can administer intrathecal narcotics for better postoperative pain control. In addition, the fetus already presents with distress. A spinal anesthestic has a faster onset which can save potentially valuable time for the fetus.

7. **Five minutes after successfully placing the spinal anesthetic, the patient's BP plummets to 60/40 mmHg and she begins to complain of severe nausea. How do you respond?**

   I would immediately place the patient in the left uterine displacement position with supplemental oxygen, open the fluids wide, assess the dermatomal level, check the FHR, and begin boluses of pressors such as phenylephrine or ephedrine.

Induction

8. **That issue is now resolved. As the surgeon begins to "test" the abdomen for sensation, the patient begins to scream loudly, complaining that she feels everything. If your decision is to convert to a general anesthetic, how will you induce the patient?**

   After preoxgenation with 100% oxygen and administering Bicitra and metoclopramide, I will perform an RSI with cricoid pressure using fentanyl, lidocaine, propofol, and succinylcholine assuming she has a normal appearing airway.

Postoperative

Postpartum hemorrhage

1. **The cesarean section was uneventful and you extubate the patient in the OR. You are now paged by the PACU nurse because the patient has abnormal vaginal bleeding. What will you do?**
   I will immediately go to the bedside and assess the patient. I will check the vital signs, urine output, mental status, acuity of blood loss, and quantify the blood loss by looking at the number of soaked vaginal pads. After informing the obstetrician, I will establish large bore IVs to support the blood pressure with crystalloids and phenylephrine, call for 4 units of PRBCs, send a STAT CBC to determine the Hb level, and have a colleague prepare the OR for possible reexploration.

2. **If the bleeding is caused by uterine atony, how would you manage?**
   First, I will actively resuscitate the patient by placing her on 100% oxygen and open the IV fluids. Second, I will carefully review the chart to see if the patient has received or is receiving any offending agents which should be stopped immediately. I will give a second dose of oxytocin and consider using Hemabate. I will avoid ergot alkaloids due to the risk of a hypertensive crisis.

Seizure

3. **This issue is resolved. A few hours later you are paged to the PACU because the patient developed a seizure. Why did this happen?**
   The risk of a preeclamptic patient developing seizures remains for 24–48 hours post delivery. Thus the patient needs to be maintained on magnesium therapy.

Postoperative hypotension

4. **On POD #1 you notice that her BP has been reading approximately 75/50 mmHg. Why do you think this is happening?**
   There are several causes of hypotension in this patient. She could be hypoxic, hypocarbic, or in a malignant arrhythmia. She may also be volume depleted secondary to her delivery and perhaps needs more IV fluids or PO fluids if tolerated. She may also still be bleeding, with resultant anemia and hypotension. Finally, her magnesium therapy, which should still be ongoing, has hypotensive side effects.

FURTHER READING

Crosby E. T. Obstetrical anaesthesia for patients with the syndrome of haemolysis, elevated liver enzymes and low platelets. *Can J Anaesth* 1991; 38(2): 227–233.

Dennis A. T. Management of pre-eclampsia: issues for anaesthetists. *Anaesthesia* 2012; 67(9): 1009–1020.

Mercier F. J. Cesarean delivery fluid management. *Curr Opin Anaesthesiol* 2012; 25(3): 286–291.

Turner J. A. Diagnosis and management of pre-eclampsia: an update. *Int J Womens Health* 2010; 30(2): 327–337.

33

Cardiac

Ruchir Gupta

Heparin

A 56 year old male is undergoing an on-pump CABG for four-vessel disease.

1a. How do you determine how much heparin to administer?
The initial dose of heparin is 3–4 mg/kg. I would thus begin with this dose and then check an ACT to determine if I have reached the therapeutic goal of 300–400 seconds. If I have not achieved that level, I would administer additional heparin.

1b. What are some adverse effects of protamine?
Protamine can cause hypotension, anaphylaxis, pulmonary hypertension, and anaphylactoid reactions.

Cardiac tamponade

You are paged to the ICU because a 75 year old patient, post aortic valve replacement, has had a steady decrease in BP. His current vital signs are BP = 101/80 mmHg, HR = 85 bpm, RR = 14, O_2 saturation 98% on 40% FiO_2. A bedside echo reveals a cardiac tamponade.

2a. What is Beck's triad?
Beck's triad is jugular venous distention, hypotension, and muffled heart sounds.

Rapid Review Anesthesiology Oral Boards, ed. Ruchir Gupta and Minh Chau Joseph Tran. Published by Cambridge University Press. © Cambridge University Press 2013.

2b. **The patient is rushed to the OR for an emergent pericardial window. Assuming the patient was extubated prior to this event, what would be your goals during induction? How do you plan on achieving them?**

Initially, I would advocate for a pericardiocentesis to be performed under local anesthesia to relieve some of the tamponade before induction and improve hemodynamics. If this is not possible, my goals during induction would be to maintain cardiac output, spontaneous ventilation, and blood pressure. With a preinduction a-line in place, I would administer midazolam, and ketamine because ketamine will increase myocardial contractility, systemic vascular resistance, and heart rate. Once the pericardial sac is opened and drained, I would administer rocuronium.

Hypertrophic cardiomyopathy

A 17 year old male football player suddenly loses consciousness during a game. Cardiac workup reveals the patient has hypertrophic cardiomyopathy (HOCM).

3a. **Do you expect this patient to have a normal ejection fraction?**

No, most patients with HOCM have an elevated EF of ~80% due to the hypercontractile state of the heart.

3b. **What cardiac abnormalities are present in a patient with HOCM?**

Usually, patients with HOCM have dynamic left ventricular outflow obstruction (due to a hypertrophied myocardium), mitral regurgitation (due to systolic anterior movement of the mitral valve), diastolic dysfunction, myocardial ischemia, and dysrhythmias.

Coarctation of the aorta

A 32 year old G1P0 presents to your labor and delivery suite for induction of labor. Her past medical history includes coarctation of the aorta.

4a. **Would you perform a regional anesthetic in this patient?**

Yes, I would. General or regional anesthesia is possible in a patient with coarctation of the aorta as long as abrupt hemodynamic changes do not occur as these can contribute to aortic dissection.

4b. **You decide on a regional technique for the case. Would you administer a spinal or an epidural?**

I would perform an epidural technique since it would allow me to slowly titrate dilute local anesthetic and prevent the abrupt sympathectomy associated with a spinal. Patients with coarctation of the aorta often have a lower pressure distal to the coarctation than proximal, so I would be wary of lowering her BP suddenly.

IABP

A 72 year old female has an intra-aortic balloon pump placed (IABP) after a long four-vessel on-pump CABG.

5a. Please describe how an IABP works.
An IABP is a counterpulsation device that sits in the aorta and works by deflating during systole, thereby reducing afterload, and inflates in diastole, thereby increasing perfusion to the coronary arteries. The net result of these actions is that there is a decrease in myocardial work and an improvement in oxygen supply to the myocardium.

5b. What are the contraindications to an IABP?
Contraindications to an IABP can be divided into relative and absolute. The absolute contraindications are severe aortic valve insufficiency, aortic dissection, and aortoiliac disease. Relative contraindications are prosthetic vascular grafts in the aorta and vascular aneurysms at the site of insertion.

Automatic internal cardiac defibrillator (AICD)

A 66 year old male presents for a laparoscopic cholecystectomy. He has an AICD in place.

6a. How would you evaluate this patient's AICD preoperatively?
I would perform a focused history and physical. I want to know his baseline cardiovascular status and the indication for the AICD. I would also want to know how often it has fired and when was the last time it was interrogated. I would also look to see if this is just an AICD or if there is a pacemaker component. I would also contact the manufacturer to see if there are any special precautions beyond what is routine for an AICD that I need to take with the specific device in the patient.

6b. How does the presence of an AICD affect your intraoperative management?
This patient is having surgery in the upper abdomen, which may come within 6 inches of the device. Depending on the AICD model, I would want to place a magnet over the AICD to inactivate it and have defibrillation pads on the patient in the event that he needs to be shocked. I would ask the surgeon to avoid electrocautery when possible and, if absolutely needed, use short bursts. I would also ask for a bipolar electrocautery and communicate frequently with the surgeon to place the magnet only when electrocautery is about to occur to minimize the amount of time that the AICD is disabled.

Cardiopulmonary bypass (CPB)

A 65 year old male is scheduled to undergo a four-vessel CABG. He has a history of diabetes, high cholesterol, and hypertension.

7a. Briefly describe the cardiopulmonary bypass machine.
The CPB machine consists of a venous reservoir where deoxygenated blood collects from the patient via a venous cannula and is then transferred to an oxygenator where it is oxygenated. The oxygenated blood is then pumped through a main pump into an arterial filter. From the arterial filter, blood is pumped through an arterial cannula back into the patient.

7b. Which type of oxygenator would you choose if you had the option for your bypass machine, a membrane or a bubble?
If I had the option, I would choose a membrane oxygenator over a bubble oxygenator because in a membrane oxygenator gas is exchanged through a semipermeable silicon membrane and is therefore less traumatic to the blood. In a bubble oxygenator, small oxygen bubbles are formed and more trauma is endured by the red blood cells.

Abdominal aortic aneurysm (AAA)

A 55 year old patient presents for open repair of an AAA.

8a. What steps can be taken to protect the patient's spinal cord during aortic cross-clamp?
To protect the spinal cord, I would (1) monitor and maintain adequate BP above and below the cross-clamp; (2) institute hypothermia; (3) use CSF drainage to optimize spinal cord perfusion pressure (SCPP), which is defined as aortic pressure minus CSF pressure or central venous pressure (whichever is greater); (4) request the surgeon to place a shunt across the cross-clamp to improve perfusion distal to the clamp; and (5) avoid vasodilators and inhalation agents that can increase ICP and thereby SCPP.

8b. Would you place an epidural for this case? Concerns?
Assuming the patient has no contraindications to a neuraxial technique such as anticoagulant therapy, back surgery, or absolute refusal of technique, I would place one. The benefits of placing one are that it allows for better postoperative pain control, improved respiratory function and pulmonary toilet postoperatively, decreased incidence of DVTs, and improved GI function. However, it can also lead to hypotension secondary to a sympathectomy, so I would be cautious in administering local anesthesia perioperatively. I would also be cognizant of the fact that this patient may develop a coagulopathy postoperatively, preventing me from removing an epidural catheter as quickly as I would like.

Down's syndrome

A 42 year old male with Down's syndrome presents for an emergency appendectomy.

9a. **What are the cardiac considerations in patients with Down's syndrome?**
Patients with Down's syndrome are at an increased risk of endocardial cushion defects, ASD, VSD, PDA, or tetralogy of Fallot. Uncorrected defects can lead to pulmonary hypertension and Eisenmenger's complex.

9b. **Why are these patients at risk for pulmonary hypertension?**
These patients are at risk for pulmonary hypertension because they are at risk of having a congenital left to right shunt which causes an increase in right-sided pressures to compensate for the shunted blood. Over time, this causes an increase in pulmonary artery pressures, progressing to pulmonary hypertension.

Bacterial endocarditis

A 21 year old female presents for a dilation and curettage. She has a history of mitral valve prolapse.

10a. **Does this patient need bacterial endocarditis prophylaxis?**
No. This patient is undergoing a GU procedure and administration of antibiotics solely to prevent infective endocarditis is no longer recommended for GU procedures.

10b. **What are the indications for bacterial endocarditis prophylaxis?**
Indications for endocarditis prophylaxis are patients with certain cardiac conditions who are undergoing certain procedures involving skin/mucosa (dental, skin, respiratory mucosa). The cardiac conditions are: prosthetic valve or prosthetic material used for repair of a valve, previous endocarditis, CHD (unrepaired cyanotic disease), completely repaired congenital heart defect with prosthetic material during first 6 months after procedure, repaired CHD with residual defect, and cardiac transplant patients who develop a valvulopathy.

FURTHER READING

Atchabahian A., Gupta R. (eds.). *The Anesthesia Guide*. New York: McGraw Hill, 2013.
Barash P. G., Cullen B. F., Stoelting R. K., Cahalan, M., Stock C. M. (eds.). *Clinical Anesthesia*, 6th edn. Philadelphia, PA: Lippincott Williams & Wilkins, 2009.
Hines R. L., Marschall K. E. (eds.). *Stoelting's Anesthesia and Co-Existing Disease*, 5th edn. Philadelphia, PA: Elsevier, 2008.

34

Obstetrics

Anita Gupta and Nicholas Weber

Cystic fibrosis (CF)

A 22 year old G1P0 female presents to the labor and delivery ward for induction. She has had no prenatal care throughout the 34 week gestation. Her PMH is significant for cystic fibrosis. The pregnancy has been uncomplicated and the patient is currently resting comfortably in bed.

1a. What are some important preoperative lab values to obtain for the CF patient?
I would want coagulation studies and serum glucose levels because CF patients often have poor hepatic function and are unable to absorb fat-soluble vitamins, e.g., vitamin K. Either of these issues may lead to coagulopathy. Many patients will be supplemented with the fat-soluble vitamins (A, D, E, K) during their pregnancy. Gestational diabetes is also common due to poor exocrine function. Oral glucose tolerance tests should be performed in each trimester, up until 30 weeks gestation.

1a. What complications may arise in a newborn with CF?
Intestinal obstruction may be the first presenting sign of CF in a newborn. Thickened meconium can accrue in utero, which may obstruct the mid-ileum. This leads to proximal dilation and bowel wall thickening. Complications such as volvulus, atresia, necrosis, perforation, meconium peritonitis, and pseudocyst formation may result.

Rapid Review Anesthesiology Oral Boards, ed. Ruchir Gupta and Minh Chau Joseph Tran. Published by Cambridge University Press. © Cambridge University Press 2013.

Multiple sclerosis (MS)

A 34 year old G3P2 female presents to labor and delivery for premature uterine contractions. She is 31 weeks pregnant and her prenatal care has been complete and unremarkable. She has a history of multiple sclerosis for the past 9 years, and has been ambulating with a cane for the last 4 years.

2a. How does pregnancy alter the disease state?

Incidence of MS relapse decreases during pregnancy, most pronounced in the third trimester, and then may increase in the first 3 months postpartum.

2b. What are the considerations when choosing an anesthetic for the parturient?

MS has implications for both regional and general anesthesia. For regional, an epidural anesthetic can be placed, but a spinal anesthetic should be avoided due to the possibility of disease exacerbation. Regarding general anesthesia, I would be hesitant to administer a depolarizing muscle relaxant because of the potential for an exaggerated release of potassium. I would instead administer an NDMR with close attention to her twitches. For either technique, I would be careful to avoid infection and fever as these are associated with an exacerbation of MS.

Epilepsy

A 26 year old G1P0 female at 39 weeks presents to labor and delivery in active labor. Her exam reveals that she is 2 cm dilated, +1, thick, and high. She has a history of epilepsy but has not been taking her medications because she has been nervous about the side effects to her child.

3a. If the mother experiences a seizure at this moment, would you treat it with Diprivan?

No. Diprivan has a high apnea potential, which is not ideal in a pregnancy state due to an anticipated difficult airway. Instead, I would administer midazolam to treat the seizures.

3b. What are the possible fetal repercussions of maternal epilepsy?

The repercussion of maternal epilepsy is that the incidence of congenital malformations such as fetal hydantoin syndrome is about two and a half times greater in neonates born to epileptic mothers. The syndrome includes intrauterine growth restriction, skull and facial abnormalities, potential cleft lip/palate, and hypoplasia of nails and digits. Also, epileptic seizures can result in fetal asphyxia depending on their severity and the progression to status epilepticus, which may have a maternal mortality of 10–25%.

Preeclampsia

A 41 year old female G1P0 who is 35 weeks pregnant has been referred to labor and delivery for induction by her obstetrician. Her blood pressure in the outpatient office was 162/102 mmHg. Also, her urine dipstick was positive for 2+ protein.

4a. Explain the spectrum of syndromes described by pregnancy-induced hypertension (PIH).

PIH describes three syndromes: preeclampsia, eclampsia, and HELLP.

Preeclampsia is defined by a triad that occurs after the 20th week of gestation. First, sustained blood pressure greater than 140/90 mmHg for mild preeclampsia and greater than 160/110 mmHg for severe preeclampsia. Second, proteinuria >2 g/day for mild and >5 g/day for severe preeclampsia. The last part of the triad is generalized edema.

Eclampsia is defined as hypertension complicated by grand mal seizures.

HELLP is a syndrome described by hypertension with hemolysis, elevated liver enzymes, and low platelets.

4b. What is the treatment for acute onset severe hypertension with preeclampsia?

As with any patient, the other vital signs must be assessed to ensure the patient is not hypoxic, hypercarbic, or in a malignant arrhythmia. If the patient is in pain, regional or IV pain medicines should be given. If the patient was anxious, I would provide verbal reassurance. If all of these potential causes were negative, I would conclude that the likely cause of the patient's hypertension is PIH. The treatment for that would be labetalol and hydralazine.

Anticoagulation in the parturient

A 24 year old female presents to the labor ward from the emergency department after her "water broke." She is 39 weeks and 2 days pregnant. She has a history of DVTs and is on anticoagulation therapy.

5a. What guidelines would you use to determine if neuraxial anesthesia is acceptable?

It depends on her anticoagulant regimen. LMWH should be held for 12 hours prior to neuraxial procedures, and held for 12 hours prior to catheter removal. If high dose LMWH is used: enoxaparin 1 mg/kg every 12 hours or 1.5 mg/kg per day, dalteparin 120 U/kg every 12 hours, dalteparin 200 U/kg, or tinzaparin 175 U/kg – then dosing should be held for 24 hours. For thienopyridine therapy, ticlopidine should be held for 14 days and clopidogrel for 7 days. ASA and NSAIDs, alone, appear to give no added risk. Coumadin is contraindicated during pregnancy because of its category X designation by the FDA.

5b. What are the additional risks of general versus neuraxial anesthesia?
General anesthesia has a mortality rate that is 16 times higher than that of neuraxial anesthesia. The major sources of mortality are attributed to hypoxia from failure to intubate the trachea and aspiration pneumonia. Additional risk factors for general anesthesia in the pregnant patient include asthma, upper respiratory tract infection, obesity, and history of difficult intubation. Apgar scores at 1 minute are lower after general anesthesia; however, no decrement in 5 minute Apgar scores has been shown.

Surgery in the pregnant patient

A 28 year old female who is 26 weeks pregnant presents to the emergency department with acute cholecystitis. Prenatal care has shown no fetal issues during the pregnancy. Fetal heart rate monitoring indicates no current fetal distress. The patient is in moderate distress and has been NPO for more than 8 hours.

6a. Surgery during which trimester carries the most risks?
Surgery during the first trimester carries the most risk because this is when organogenesis occurs. In addition, the first trimester carries the highest risk for spontaneous abortions.

6b. Do you still need to perform an RSI on this patient knowing that she has been NPO for more than 8 hours?
Yes. I would still perform an RSI on this patient. There are several factors that decrease the GI transit time for this pregnant woman: gravid uterus, sympathetic nervous system > parasympathetic nervous system from the painful cholecystitis, and narcotics given to the patient in the ER to treat the pain.

Labor epidural

A 23 year old G1P0 female requests a labor epidural for vaginal delivery. The obstetricians tell you that the patient has been compliant with all of her prenatal care, and she has had no obstetric issues. While completing your history and physical she denied any past medical or surgical history.

7a. What are the absolute and relative contraindications to epidural analgesia?
Absolute: Patient refusal, sepsis with hemodynamic instability, uncorrected hypovolemia with ongoing hemorrhage, coagulopathy.

Relative: Elevated intracranial pressure, prior back injury with neurologic deficit, progressive neurologic disease e.g., multiple sclerosis, chronic back pain, localized infection at the injection site.

7b. What physiologic changes are expected with an epidural anesthesia?

The physiologic changes that are expected are: (1) sympathectomy resulting in reduced afterload and a decrease in blood pressure, with possible reflex tachycardia; (2) vasodilation that may also decrease core temperature leading to shivering; (3) bladder distention and contraction of the bowel caused by unopposed parasympathetics; (4) decreased awareness of the motions of breathing, which may lead to the feeling of dyspnea.

Uterine atony

A 35 year old female G6P5 is currently undergoing a C-section for failure to progress. The patient is being managed in the operating room with a working epidural and she appears comfortable. A healthy baby was delivered. Immediately after removal of the placenta you estimate the blood loss to be greater than 1000 mL.

8a. What are the risk factors for uterine atony?

Uterine atony is failure of the uterus to contract after delivery. Atony is associated with overdistention of the uterus. Thus, the risk factors for uterine atony are multiparity, polyhydramnios, chorioamnionitis, augmented labor, large infants, and retained placenta.

8b. How is uterine atony managed?

Initially, bimanual compression and uterine massage is performed by the obstetric team. Pharmacologically, oxytocin is the first line, then intramuscular methylergonovine. For refractory uterine atony, 15-methylprostaglandin F2-alpha may be given intramyometrially or intramuscularly. Coagulation factors may need replacement. Uterine bleed refractory to pharmacologic measures is then controlled by ligation of the hypogastric arteries. The final measure is hysterectomy.

Aortic stenosis

A 24 year old, full term female with congenital aortic stenosis is requesting an epidural for labor analgesia. Pelvic ultrasound has revealed IUGR. The patient has not received prenatal care, and she is uncomfortable from her contractions.

9a. What are the normal hemodynamic changes of pregnancy?

The hemodynamic changes of pregnancy are associated with an increase in intravascular fluid volume. Anemia of pregnancy is a consequence of plasma volume increasing by 45% and erythrocyte volume increasing by 20%. Cardiac output increases by 50% by the 3rd trimester and by 80% postpartum. Stroke volume is increased by 30% and heart rate is increased by 15–25%. Systemic vascular resistance decreases by 15%. As a consequence of these shifts, mean arterial blood pressure may decrease by 15 mmHg, largely due to a decrease in diastolic blood pressure.

9b. **Describe the hemodynamics of fixed aortic outflow obstruction and the theoretical issues that are complicated by neuraxial anesthesia.**
Coronary perfusion pressure (CPP) is defined as aortic diastolic pressure (aortDBP) minus left ventricular end-diastolic pressure (LVEDP). In aortic stenosis, the LVEDP is elevated, causing a decrease in CPP. Thus, to maintain a CPP it is important to maintain the aortic BP, which correlates to MAP. The complication with neuraxial anesthesia is that it results in vasodilation and a decrease in MAP. Thus, to maintain CPP, one must prehydrate the patient and have pressors on standby to correct any sudden drops in BP.

von Willebrand's disease (vWD)

A 31 year old female 37 weeks pregnant presents to labor and delivery with blood seeping through her pants. She says she has von Willebrand's disease. Previous hemoglobin levels have been in the normal range.

10a. **Describe vWD.**
Von Willebrand's disease is a qualitative and/or quantitative defect in vWF which stabilizes factor VIII, thereby promoting clotting. Type 1 is the most common and is believed to be due to a decrease in actual vWF. Most patients with this type are asymptomatic. Type 2 is due to a qualitative defect in vWF and again is not clinically significant. Type 3 is the most severe form and is due to a virtual absence of vWF resulting in mucosal hemorrhage, hemarthrosis, and hematomas.

10b. **What can be used to attenuate the bleeding in this patient?**
Depending on the type of vWD, different treatment modalities are available. For type 1, pregnancy itself will increase circulating levels of vWF. Also, DDAVP is used to stimulate release of vWF from endothelial cells and is helpful with type 1 patients. For types 2 and 3 or if the patient is a nonresponder to DDAVP, cryoprecipitate, FFP, or factor VIII-vWF concentrates (Humate P) may be used.

FURTHER READING

Barash P., Cullen B., Stoelting R. *Clinical Anesthesia*, 5th edn. Philadelphia, PA: Lippincott Williams & Wilkins, 2006.

Devonshire V., Duquette P., Dwosh E., Guimond C. The immune system and hormones: review and relevance to pregnancy and contraception in women with MS. *Int MS J* 2003; 10: 44–50.

Donaldson J. Neurologic emergencies in pregnancy. *Obstet Gynecol* 1997; 177: 1–7.

Duke J. *Anesthesia Secrets*, 3rd edn. Mosby Elsevier, 2006.

Edenborough F. P., Stableforth D. E., Webb A. K., Mackenzie W. E., Smith D. L. Outcome of pregnancy in women with cystic fibrosis. *Thorax* 1995; 50: 170–174.

Goss C. H., Rubenfeld G. D., Otto K., Aitken M. L. The effect of pregnancy on survival in women with cystic fibrosis. *Chest* 2003; 124: 1460–1468.

Hughes S., Levinson G., Rosen M. *Shinder and Levinson's Anesthesia for Obstetrics*, 4th edn. Philadelphia, PA: Lippincott Williams & Wilkins, 2002.

Irish M., Reynolds M. *Surgical aspects of cystic fibrosis and meconium ileus*. Medscape Reference, 2011.

Mygind K. I., Mogens D., Christiansen J. Phenytoin and phenobarbitone plasma clearance during pregnancy. *Acta Neurol Scand* 1976; 54: 160–166.

Reed A., Yudkowitz F. *Clinical Cases in Anesthesia*, 3rd edn. Philadelphia, PA: Elsevier Churchill Livingstone, 2005.

Stoelting R., Dierdorf S. *Anesthesia and Co-Existing Disease*, 4th edn. Philadelphia, PA: Churchill Livingstone Elsevier, 2002.

Stoelting R., Miller R. *Basics of Anesthesia*, 5th edn. Philadelphia, PA: Churchill Livingstone Elsevier, 2007.

Verma A., Das M., Ahluwalia A., et al. Pregnancy and cystic fibrosis. *Cystic Fibrosis Trust*. cysticfibrosismedicine.com, 2004.

Pediatrics

Ruchir Gupta, Monique Cadogan, and Barbara Vickers

Malignant hyperthermia

A 5 year old boy presents to your ambulatory surgery center for a tonsillectomy and adenoidectomy. His father tells you that the patient's mother died of a "fever" during surgery.

1a. Would you delay the case to perform a muscle biopsy on the child?
No. Based on the information given, I would treat this child as MH susceptible and avoid all triggering agents. Thus, a muscle biopsy would not change my management. In addition, the cost and discomfort associated with the biopsy may not be tolerated by the patient and family. This surgery can be safely executed with nontriggering agents and a muscle biopsy is not needed.

1b. Would you insist this case be performed at a pediatric hospital as opposed to an ambulatory surgical center?
No. This surgery can be safely conducted in an ambulatory surgical center provided that the necessary precautions are taken: avoidance of triggering agents, availability of an MH cart, and availability of supportive, resuscitative, and monitoring equipment.

King–Denborough syndrome

An 8 year old female with a history of King–Denborough syndrome presents for an emergency appendectomy. She has never had surgery before.

2a. What are the principal anesthetic considerations in this patient?
The principal anesthetic consideration in this patient is that she is susceptible to malignant hyperthermia because of her history of King–Denborough

Rapid Review Anesthesiology Oral Boards, ed. Ruchir Gupta and Minh Chau Joseph Tran. Published by Cambridge University Press. © Cambridge University Press 2013.

syndrome. Thus, all triggering agents should be avoided and the MH cart should be readily available.

2b. What steps will you take to reduce the chance of this patient developing malignant hyperthermia?

There are several things that I will do to reduce the risk. First, I will remove all triggering agents such as succinylcholine and volatile anesthetic vaporizers from the room. I will also flush out my anesthesia machine with 100% O_2 to remove any residual gases. Next, I will review the contents of my MH cart, making sure the drugs are all up to date and have not expired. Then, I will have a team meeting with the nurses, surgeons, and any residents/fellows to delegate roles if an MH episode did occur. Finally, I will inform the PACU that an MH-susceptible patient is about to have surgery and they should reserve a bed in the ICU in the event an emergent transfer is needed. If I am working in a hospital that does not have a pediatric ICU, I would also contact the nearest tertiary care center and request to have a bed available in case the patient needs to be emergently transferred.

CHARGE syndrome

A 5 year old Mexican male is scheduled for a cochlear implant. The child was brought to the US by a religious mission that is funding his care. He has a history of CHARGE syndrome.

3a. What are the airway considerations for a patient with CHARGE syndrome?

Patients with CHARGE syndrome commonly have a cleft lip and palate. In addition, they may also present with micrognathia, laryngomalacia, subglottic stenosis, recurrent laryngeal nerve palsy, tracheomalacia, and tracheoesophageal fistula. Care must be taken to identify which of these abnormalities are present and difficult airway equipment should be on standby along with an ENT surgeon for an emergent tracheostomy.

3b. Will you insist on an echocardiogram prior to taking this patient to the OR?

Yes, I would want an echocardiogram in this patient because up to 75% of patients with CHARGE syndrome have concomitant cardiac defects. These defects can be simple but can also be very complex, such as tetralogy of Fallot.

Treacher Collins syndrome

A 4 year old patient with a history of Treacher Collins syndrome presents for an emergency appendectomy.

4a. What are the major differences between the Treacher Collins and the Pierre Robin syndromes?
Both syndromes are associated with micrognathia and difficult airways, but Pierre Robin syndrome is also known for glossoptosis. In addition, while cardiac defects occur with increased frequency in both populations, other congenital defects are more common with Treacher Collins syndrome than with Pierre Robin syndrome.

4b. How are you going to secure the airway in this patient?
These patients are known to have difficult airways. Thus, I will have the difficult airway cart in the room, with the neck prepped and draped with a tracheostomy kit open and ready. Then, I will administer PO midazolam and perform a sedated fiberoptic intubation while maintaining spontaneous ventilations. If the patient remains uncooperative, I will administer titrating doses of ketamine and glycopyrrolate while maintaining spontaneous ventilations. Once the patient is sedated, I will use my fiberoptic scope to visualize the vocal cords and insert the ETT.

Tetralogy of Fallot

A 3 year old male patient is scheduled for a cardiac catheterization. The patient's mother states that the child frequently "turns blue."

5a. What may explain this finding?
When venous blood bypasses the lungs and returns to the systemic circulation (right-to-left shunting), patients are at risk of cyanosis.

5b. How does a right-to-left cardiac shunt impact intravenous induction? Inhalational induction?
A patient with a right-to-left shunt would have a faster intravenous induction and a slower inhalation induction. To reduce further intraoperative right-to-left intracardiac shunting, higher systemic vascular resistance is utilized.

Pyloric stenosis

A 3 week old female with pyloric stenosis requires a laparoscopic pyloromyotomy. She is full term and otherwise healthy.

6a. **What would you expect her chemistry panel to show?**
I would expect a hypochloremic, hypokalemic, metabolic alkalosis secondary to persistent vomiting. In extreme cases where the dehydration is severe, this may progress to a metabolic acidemia secondary to hypoperfusion.

6b. **Assuming the patient is medically optimized, how would you induce this patient?**
Due to the severe risk for aspiration, the stomach needs to be decompressed either via an NG or OG tube in the lateral, supine, and prone positions to remove as much of the gastric contents as possible. After preoxygenating the child with 100% O_2 and atropine to prevent a vagal response to direct laryngoscopy, I will perform a rapid sequence induction with propofol and rocuronium.

Airway management

You are paged by the PACU nurse for a 4 year old female who following tonsillectomy and adenoidectomy has been vomiting blood. Her BP is 63/32 mmHg while supine, heart rate 134 bpm, and respiratory rate 24.

7a. **Once the child is brought back to the OR, how will you induce this patient?**
For induction, I will choose agents that provide the best hemodynamic support given this patient's unstable vital signs and full stomach status. After preoxygenating with 100% O_2, I will perform a rapid sequence intubation with cricoid pressure using ketamine and rocuronium.

7b. **Your resident suggests using succinylcholine because this patient's airway needs to be rapidly secured due to her bleeding tonsil. How do you respond?**
I would inform the resident that while the airway is concerning, rocuronium in adequate doses can provide similar paralytic onset time to succinylcholine. Succinylcholine carries the additional risk of precipitating malignant hyperthermia in this patient if there were an undiagnosed myopathy. Thus, the risks of succinylcholine outweigh the benefits.

Down's syndrome – preoperative evaluation

A 2 year old male with Down's syndrome presents for a left inguinal hernia repair.

8a. **What are your preoperative concerns in this patient?**
Down's syndrome has clinical manifestations in just about every major organ system. My concerns are as follows:

Airway: These patients often have macroglossia and subglottic stenosis, both of which contribute to a potentially difficult airway.

GI: If this patient has duodenal atresia, I would treat him as a full stomach.

Cardiac: These patients often have coexisting endocardial cushion defects. I would want to know what coexisting cardiac defects he has since this will affect my choice of induction/maintenance agents. A baseline echo might be warranted.

Neuro: These patients can have atlantoaxial subluxation. Thus, I would want to maintain this patient's neck in the neutral position and avoid any maneuvers that can strain or place pressure on the neck.

Respiratory: Obstructive airway disease is often present in these patients and they are more prone to snoring and apnea. These patients are also at increased risk for infection, vision loss, and hearing loss.

8b. **During the neurologic evaluation, you notice the patient has a positive Babinski sign. Does this concern you?**

Yes, it does. A positive Babinski sign argues strongly for the possibility of neurologic compromise in this patient, most likely secondary to the atlantoaxial subluxation. I would inform the parents that such a condition increases this patient's risk for perioperative neurologic compromise. It would be wise to reschedule this elective case once the patient has been evaluated by a neurologist.

Down's syndrome – intraoperative management

A 4 year old patient with Down's syndrome presents for a tonsillectomy and adenoidectomy.

9a. **How would you secure the airway in this patient?**

Before the patient is brought into the OR, I will make sure the emergency airway cart is in the room as well as the ENT surgeon. After a careful airway exam, I will perform an inhalational induction with oxygen and sevoflurane. Once the child is mask induced and an IV established, I will keep the neck neutral and avoid neck extension during the direct laryngoscopy.

9b. **The patient had a tetralogy of Fallot repaired at 2 years of age. Does this patient need infective endocarditis (IE) prophylaxis?**

No. IE prophylaxis is only indicated in patients with certain cardiac conditions who are undergoing dental procedures. IE prophylaxis is warranted in patients with a history of prosthetic valve or prosthetic material used for repair of a valve, previous endocarditis, congenital heart disease (unrepaired cyanotic disease), completely repaired congenital heart defect with prosthetic material during first 6 months after procedure, repaired CHD with residual defect, and cardiac transplant patients who develop a valvulopathy.

Omphalocele

A 5 kg, 1 day old male presents for closure of an omphalocele.

10a. What are the key differences between an omphalocele and a gastroschisis?

There are several differences between an omphalocele and a gastroschisis. First, an omphalocele is usually located within the umbilical cord whereas a gastroschisis is to the right of it. Second, an omphalocele has a membranous sac covering it, whereas in gastroschisis there is no covering and the viscera is exposed. Finally, an omphalocele is associated with several conditions including Beckwith–Wiedemann syndrome, CHD, trisomy 13, 18, or 21, and pentalogy of Cantrell. Gastroschisis, by contrast, is associated mainly with prematurity and intestinal atresia.

10b. At the end of the procedure, the patient begins to desaturate as the abdomen is being closed. How will you respond?

Based on the information given, it seems likely that the patient is desaturating due to impaired pulmonary compliance from increased abdominal pressure from the wound closure. Thus, after making sure the other vitals were stable, I would immediately ask the surgeon to open the wound and relieve the abdominal pressure. A staged closure where only superficial layers are initially closed would then have to occur.

FURTHER READING

Barash P. G., Cullen B. F., Stoelting R. K., Cahalan M., Stock, C. M. (eds.). *Clinical Anesthesia*, 6th edn. Philadelphia, PA: Lippincott Williams & Wilkins, 2009.

Hines R. L., Marschall K. E. (eds.). *Stoelting's Anesthesia and Co-Existing Disease*, 5th edn. Philadelphia, PA: Elsevier, 2008.

Practice advisory for the perioperative management of patients with cardiac implantable electronic devices: pacemakers and implantable cardioverter-defibrillators. An updated report by the American Society of Anesthesiologists task force on perioperative management of patients with cardiac implantable electronic devices. *Anesthesiology* 2011; 114: 247–261.

Touloukian R. J., Higgins E. The spectrum of serum electrolytes in hypertrophic pyloric stenosis. *J Pediatric Surg* 1983; 18(4): 394–397.

36

Neuro

Ruchir Gupta

Cerebral aneurysm

A 55 year old male with a history of CAD presents for emergency clipping of a partially ruptured cerebral aneurysm. On physical exam, he has a Mallampati IV airway and limited neck movement secondary to a previous cervical fusion.

1a. The surgeon asks you to perform a slow controlled induction to avoid life-threatening HTN in this patient which could cause aneurysmal rupture. How do you respond?

I would inform the surgeon that this patient is not a candidate for a slow controlled induction because of his difficult airway. I would also tell the surgeon that to ensure the patient has stable hemodynamics during the awake intubation, I will perform airway blocks (superior laryngeal/recurrent laryngeal), administer nebulized lidocaine, have a preinduction a-line with an esmolol drip attached to emergently treat any rise in BP during the intubation.

1b. During the dissection of the aneurysm, the patient's BP is 100/60 mmHg. The surgeon asks you to lower the BP further to aid in the dissection. How do you respond?

My concern in this patient is to maintain a BP that is sufficiently low to perfuse the coronary arteries without inducing myocardial ischemia. Thus, I will look at the current BP and corresponding EKG to rule out signs of myocardial ischemia. Then, I will begin to administer nitroglycerin or esmolol infusion slowly while looking at my EKG for any signs of ischemia. I will also ask the surgeon to place a temporary clip on the feeding vessel to lower the amount of blood entering the aneurysm.

Rapid Review Anesthesiology Oral Boards, ed. Ruchir Gupta and Minh Chau Joseph Tran. Published by Cambridge University Press. © Cambridge University Press 2013.

Intracranial tumor

A 67 year old female presents for resection of an intracranial tumor.

2a. What are the components of ICP?
ICP is composed of cerebral tissue, CSF, and cerebral blood volume.

2b. How would you determine if this patient has an elevated ICP preoperatively?
Preoperatively, I would perform a focused history and physical. From the history, I will ask the patient if she has any nausea or vomiting, weakness in any part of her body, or any headaches. From the physical, I will want to know if there have been any changes in mentation from baseline. Any evidence of somnolence will strongly argue for an elevated ICP. I will also examine for the presence of papilledema and focal neurologic deficits such as nerve palsy or muscle weakness.

Autonomic hyperreflexia

A surgeon wishes to perform incision and drainage of a chronic heel ulcer on a paraplegic patient with a T4 spinal cord transection.

3a. The surgeon asks you to administer 2 mg of midazolam as the patient has no sensation below the level of the lesion. How do you respond?
I would inform the surgeon that administering midazolam would not be sufficient anesthesia for this patient because this patient is at high risk for autonomic hyperreflexia. Autonomic hyperreflexia can only be prevented by removing the surgical stimulus or administering a deep general anesthetic so as to prevent the patient from feeling the surgical stimulus.

3b. What is the pathogenesis of autonomic hyperreflexia?
Autonomic hyperreflexia results from a stimulus below the level of transection causing sympathetically mediated HTN, bradycardia, sweating, and flushing above the lesion.

Cerebral vasospasm

A 70 year old male underwent aneurysm clipping for a subarachnoid hemorrhage 1 day ago and has been in the neurosurgical ICU overnight intubated and sedated.

4a. What are the major postoperative concerns you would have for this patient?
These patients are at high risk for the development of seizures, so antiseizure prophylaxis is given. They are also at high risk for rebleeding, so BP must be

controlled. Hydrocephalus is also a concern and is treated with ventricular drainage. Finally, vasospasm is common typically from days 3–15 post-bleed and daily sonographic exams must be performed to detect vasospasm.

4b. What is meant by the term "triple H" therapy?
Triple H therapy refers to hypertension, hypervolemia, and hemodilution. This therapy is indicated as treatment for cerebral vasospasm.

TURP syndrome

A 54 year old male is undergoing a transurethral retrograde prostatectomy (TURP) under spinal anesthesia.

5a. What steps can you take to minimize this patient's risk of developing TURP syndrome?
To minimize the risk of TURP syndrome, I can make sure the height gradient between the irrigation fluid and the patient is minimized to reduce the hydrostatic pressure, limit the duration of the procedure, and maintain verbal contact with the patient throughout the procedure.

5b. Midway through the case the patient becomes confused and tachycardic. You intubate and place an arterial line. A STAT Na level comes back at 121 mEq/L. Will you administer hypertonic saline?
No. Correction of Na must be gradual so as to prevent central pontine myelinolysis. At 121 mEq/L, I would begin with securing the airway, restricting fluid, administering furosemide, and evaluating for EKG changes. If the condition continues to deteriorate and his Na continues to decrease, I will consider administering hypertonic saline.

Pituitary tumor

A 45 year old male presents for resection of a growth hormone secreting pituitary tumor.

6a. What are your preoperative concerns regarding his condition?
My concerns regarding his condition are that he may display signs of acromegaly which would make it difficult to secure the airway. Also, this patient may have glottic stenosis, necessitating a smaller diameter ETT with proper tests for a leak to ensure there is no compression of the cuff on the tracheal mucosa. My non-airway concerns would be an increased incidence of CAD, HTN, OSA, and insulin resistance in this patient. I would probe to see which of these conditions the patient has and how severe an effect they have had on his organ systems so that I can tailor my anesthesia accordingly.

6b. **How will you secure the airway?**

Given this patient's risk for a difficult airway, I would want to perform an awake fiberoptic intubation in this patient. I will begin by administering 4% nebulized lidocaine, glycopyrrolate, and small, titrating doses of a benzodiazepine prior to placing the scope.

ECT

You are asked to provide anesthesia for a 39 year old male with bipolar disorder. Upon reviewing this patient's medication list, you notice he has been on lithium.

7a. **Will you delay the case?**

Yes. Lithium must be withheld for 36–72 hours or else it may cause a prolongation of the seizure with resulting dysrhythmias or delirium.

7b. **On further questioning, the patient tells you that recently he has been urinating significantly more than he has in the past. Could this be related to his lithium?**

Yes. Lithium therapy is associated with diabetes insipidus. Treatment of lithium-induced diabetes insipidus is cessation or reduction of the offending agent.

Hyponatremia

A 34 year old male underwent an open reduction of a right humerus after a severe motorcycle accident in which he wasn't wearing a helmet. A head CT scan reveals a small stable subdural hematoma. On POD #2 his Na level is 127 mEq/L.

8a. **What is the mechanism of action of SIADH?**

SIADH results from unregulated release of antidiuretic hormone (ADH), which acts on the distal convoluted tubule and the collecting duct to reabsorb water, not solute. The result of this is retention of water with a dilution of solute, leading to hyponatremia, decreased serum osmolarity, increased urine osmolarity, and decreased urine production.

8b. **How can you distinguish SIADH from cerebral salt wasting syndrome (CSWS)?**

Clinically, one would see hypovolemia in CSWS and euvolemia or hypervolemia in SIADH. In terms of lab studies, the urine osmolarity is high in SIADH and low to normal in CSWS. Furthermore, polyuria is seen in CSWS whereas urinary output is decreased in SIADH.

Peripheral neuropathy

A 47 year old female complains of persistent left little finger weakness one week after her laparoscopic cholecystectomy.

9a. How will you evaluate this patient?

I would perform a focused history and physical. From the history, I would want to know when the symptoms began, whether they are getting better or worse, whether there is any pain accompanying the weakness, and whether there is also a sensory component. From the physical, I would examine the area for signs of infection or inflammation, assess muscle strength, and clearly delineate the area of the sensory loss with a marking pen.

9b. Assuming this was an ulnar nerve injury secondary to malpositioning, how would you treat this?

I would begin treatment with conservative measures as well as follow-up visits because most of these injuries are self-limiting. If the symptoms persist or worsen, I would order EMG studies and request a neurology consult.

Multiple sclerosis

A 38 year old female with multiple sclerosis presents for a right hemicolectomy.

10a. What precautions would you take to prevent exacerbation of her MS symptoms?

To prevent exacerbation, I would avoid any increase in body temperature, whether iatrogenic or from an infection. I would exercise judicious use of antibiotics, and ensure that my Bair Hugger is not delivering too much warm air to the patient. I will also avoid a spinal anesthetic in this patient because spinal techniques have been implicated in exacerbation of symptoms. In the postoperative period, I will perform periodic neurologic checks and also ensure that the patient does not experience any rise in temperature.

10b. Can this patient have neuraxial anesthesia for this case?

Yes, this patient can have an epidural neuraxial block. For reasons that are unclear, patients with MS who received spinal anesthesia experienced an exacerbation of symptoms whereas those with an epidural or peripheral nerve blocks did not. It is believed that this may be due to the fact that MS renders the spinal cord more susceptible to the toxic effects of local anesthetics.

FURTHER READING

Atchabahian A., Gupta R. (eds.). *The Anesthesia Guide*. New York: McGraw-Hill Publishing, 2013.

Cottrell J. E., Young W. L. (eds.). *Cottrell's Neuroanesthesia*, 5th edn. Elsevier Health Sciences, 2010.

37

Pain management

Ruchir Gupta

Pain onset

A 35 year old female injured her shoulder during an ice skating accident. She presents today with persistent right arm pain.

1a. What is the mechanism of peripheral nerve sensitization to pain? Central nervous sensitization?

Tissue damage results in the release of inflammatory mediators, which sensitize peripheral nerves. Central sensitization refers to the increased synaptic efficacy in the spinal cord caused by intense painful stimuli or nerve damage. As a result, this increased synaptic transmission causes patients to have a lower threshold for pain, an increased sensation to otherwise mild pain, and increased sensitivity to pain in non-injured areas.

1b. What is meant by allodynia?

Allodynia is a pain sensation caused by a stimulus which does not normally provoke pain. This is different from hyperalgesia, an exaggerated reaction to a stimulus which is normally painful.

Chronic pain

You are consulted on a 67 year old patient with end-stage pancreatic cancer, now in hospice care. The primary care resident claims that multiple pain therapies have been attempted, but the patient continues to be in extreme pain all the time.

2a. How will you evaluate this patient?

I will perform a focused history and physical. From the history, I will want to know where the pain is located, its intensity, radiation, and coexisting

Rapid Review Anesthesiology Oral Boards, ed. Ruchir Gupta and Minh Chau Joseph Tran. Published by Cambridge University Press. © Cambridge University Press 2013.

symptoms. I will also want to know which medicines have been administered and what effect they have had on the pain. If the patient had any interventional pain management techniques, I will also want to know about that. From the physical, I will examine the patient to assess where exactly the pain is located. Though I am told this is from pancreatic cancer, I will also evaluate for other causes of the pain such as inflammation from another cause at the site of the pain. Finally, I will look at imaging studies such as a CT scan of the abdomen to see if surgical debulking is a possibility.

2b. Will you use opioids to treat this patient's pain?

Yes. It appears that the patient is suffering from breakthrough pain despite multiple pain modalities (step 3 of the WHO pain ladder). I would administer opioids to acutely reduce her pain. Once her pain is under control, I will consult a pain specialist to develop a short- to intermediate-term pain plan for this patient.

Complex regional pain syndrome (CRPS) type 1

A patient is referred to your outpatient pain clinic for evaluation of a complex regional pain syndrome (CRPS).

3a. What is complex regional pain syndrome?

CRPS is a disease resulting from the dysregulation of the CNS which leads to pain, burning, swelling, and changes in skin color and temperature. CRPS usually follows a relatively minor trauma such as contusion, sprain, fracture, or dislocation.

3b. How would you determine if this patient has CRPS 1 or 2?

CRPS types 1 and 2 are distinguished mainly by the etiology. Whereas CRPS 1 can result from injury to any part of the body, CRPS type 2 results from injury to a nerve bundle. The pain onset is usually immediate and is associated with allodynia, hyperpathia, and vasomotor changes.

Stellate ganglion

You are performing a stellate ganglion block on a 32 year old female who developed CRPS in her right upper extremity.

4a. Where is the stellate ganglion located?

Stellate ganglion is located at the level of C7 (7th cervical vertebra), anterior to the transverse process of C7, anterior to the neck of the first rib, and just below the subclavian artery.

4b. What are the possible complications associated with a stellate ganglion block?

Complications of stellate ganglion blocks are: intravascular injection, subarachnoid injection, hematoma, pneumothorax, brachial plexus block, hoarseness due to recurrent laryngeal nerve injury, and epidural block.

Myofascial pain

A 48 year old female has been receiving trigger point injections in her upper back regions, containing steroid and local anesthetic for myofascial pain.

5a. What are trigger points?

Trigger points are areas in the skeletal muscle that are hyperirritable. Often times, palpable nodules in taut bands of muscle fibers are present with focal point tenderness. Injection of local anesthetic at these points is the mainstay of treatment in patients with myofascial pain.

5b. How does the TENS therapy work?

There are different proposed mechanisms for how TENS works. Inhibition of pain signals at presynaptic levels is one mechanism. Another mechanism involves electrical impulse stimulation which causes the release of endogenous substances involved in pain control.

Opioids

A 36 year old G1P0 female is on chronic methadone therapy. She is currently 36 weeks pregnant.

6a. Should you stop her methadone to prevent neonatal narcotic dependency?

No, I would not because patients on chronic methadone therapy risk preterm labor, fetal distress, or fetal demise if abruptly discontinued. In fact, it has been suggested to increase the methadone dose during the third trimester since maternal volume of distribution is increased leading to a dilutional effect of the methadone.

6b. What are your concerns for her newborn?

I am concerned that the newborn is at risk for neonatal abstinence syndrome (NAS). This syndrome manifests as increased sweating, nasal stuffiness, fever, temperature instability, tachypnea, and mottling of the skin, tremors, irritability, increased wakefulness, high-pitched crying, myoclonus, hypertonicity and hyperactive reflexes, yawning, sneezing, and skin excoriation due to excessive rubbing. A small percentage may develop seizures. These patients may also have poor feeding, uncoordinated and constant sucking, vomiting or regurgitation, loose or watery stools, and dehydration.

Local anesthetic toxicity

Shortly after injecting 0.5% bupivacaine for a spinal anesthetic, the patient begins to complain of nausea and light-headedness.

7a. How will you respond?
I will immediately lay the patient supine and administer 100% O_2 while looking at her vital signs to make sure she is not hypoxic or in a malignant arrhythmia. I will open my fluids wide and administer boluses of a vasopressor such as ephedrine or phenylephrine. Because IV injection of bupivacaine is associated with non-resuscitatable cardiac arrest, I will call for the code cart and call for help as a precautionary measure.

7b. Despite your intervention the patient develops cardiac arrest. What is the treatment for bupivacaine-induced cardiac toxicity and what is the dose you would use?
I would use 20% intralipid at a dose of 1.5 mL/kg IV over 1 minute followed by an infusion of 0.25 mL/kg. If the symptoms did not improve, I would repeat the bolus at 1–2 times the initial dose with an infusion of 0.5 mL/kg.

Cancer pain

A 72 year old patient with end-stage pancreatic cancer presents for a celiac plexus block.

8a. What are the side effects and complications of a celiac plexus block?
Side effects and complications of a celiac plexus block include life-threatening hypotension secondary to the sympathectomy, hemorrhage from vascular injury, abdominal cramping and diarrhea from unopposed parasympathetic action, organ injury, local anesthetic toxicity, paraplegia from damage to the artery of Adamkiewicz, and neuronal injury.

8b. If this patient had uterine cancer rather than pancreatic cancer, which block would you perform?
In the case of uterine cancer, a superior hypogastric plexus block is used because the pain arises from the pelvic viscera.

Post-amputation pain

A 26 year old male had a left below-the-knee amputation performed 6 weeks ago following a motor cycle accident. The patient continues to complain of pain in the left toes.

9a. Your resident wants to call a psychiatry consult because the patient is complaining of pain in areas that no longer exist. Do you agree?

No, I would not rush to call a psychiatry consult. This patient may be experiencing phantom limb pain which is relatively common in post amputee patients. Phantom limb pain is a complex syndrome with a wide array of sequelae ranging from severe pain to tingling and itching. Several theories have been advanced regarding the neurologic basis with no absolute consensus.

9b. What is the treatment for phantom limb pain?

There is no absolutely satisfactory treatment for this syndrome. Current treatment modalities include spinal cord stimulation, heat application, vibration therapy, acupuncture, physical therapy, hypnosis, biofeedback, and medications such as antidepressants, anticonvulsants, beta blockers, and sodium channel blockers.

Lower back pain and sciatica

A 62 year old construction worker presents to the interventional pain clinic with chronic lower back pain.

10a. How would you evaluate the patient?

I would perform a focused history and physical. From the history, I would want to know where the pain is, how severe on a scale of 1–10, with or without radiation, any exacerbating/alleviating factors, and what treatment modalities he has attempted and what were those outcomes. From the physical, I would want to examine his back, looking for gross signs of inflammation (rubor, calor, dolor) as well as any gross deformities. I will also look to assess if the pain is tender to palpation.

10b. An MRI ordered by his primary care physician shows an L5–S1 disc degeneration. He has been on NSAIDs, opioids, and physical therapy with minimal relief. Recently the pain has been radiating down his right leg. What treatment options would you offer this patient?

I would review with him his past medications and assess if the maximum dose of opioids as well as non-opioid drugs have been given and if not, what side effects, if any, prevented the continued use of those drugs. In terms of procedures, I would discuss with the patient the possibility of a lumbar epidural steroid injection to place medicine in the epidural space. If the symptoms were unilateral, a transforaminal approach could be used.

FURTHER READING

Argoff C. E., McCleane, G. (eds.). *Pain Management Secrets*, 3rd edn. Philadelphia, PA: Mosby Elsevier, 2009.

Fishman S. M., Ballantyne J. C., Rathmell J. P. (eds.). *Bonica's Management of Pain*, 4th edn. Philadelphia, PA: Lippincott Williams & Wilkins, 2009.

Miller R. D., Eriksson L. I., Fleisher L. A., Wiener-Kornish J. P., Young W. L. (eds.). *Miller's Anesthesia*, 7th edn. Philadelphia, PA: Churchill Livingstone Elsevier, 2010.

Warfield C. A., Bajwa Z. H. (eds.). *Principles and Practice of Pain Medicine*, 2nd edn. New York, NY: McGraw-Hill Medical Publishing Division, 2004.

38

Neuraxial and anticoagulation

Ruchir Gupta

Neuraxial in COPD patient

A 68 year old COPD patient with a 50 pack year smoking history presents for a cystoscopy.

1a. What is the best anesthetic technique for this patient?
I would choose an epidural technique. The benefits of an epidural are avoidance of intubation and ventilatory support, fewer DVTs, better postoperative pain control, fewer systemic side effects from opioids, and quicker ambulation.

1b. What information would you require prior to performing a neuraxial technique in this patient?
I would want to know if this patient has any coagulopathies, is on any anticoagulant medication, if he has any history of nerve injuries, any back surgeries with or without instrumentation, and any problems with any neuraxial technique he may have undergone in the past.

Heparin with PCEA

You are paged by a nurse on the medical floor to remove an epidural catheter in a patient with a PCEA.

2a. How long since the last heparin dose must you wait before removing the catheter?
It depends on the type of heparin. If it is unfractionated subcutaneous heparin, there is no delay. If it is IV unfractionated, then I would wait 2–4 hours. If it is LMWH low dose QD dosing, then I would wait 12 hours, low dose BID dosing, I would have removed the catheter prior to initiating treatment, LMWH high dose, I would wait 24 hours.

Rapid Review Anesthesiology Oral Boards, ed. Ruchir Gupta and Minh Chau Joseph Tran. Published by Cambridge University Press. © Cambridge University Press 2013.

2b. How long will you require the heparin for this patient to be held after you remove the catheter?

I would ask for it to be held for 1 hour if it is IV unfractionated heparin and 2 hours if it is LMWH, regardless of dose.

Neuraxial in CAD

A 55 year old female with three cardiac stents presents for a right knee replacement. She is currently on Plavix and ASA for her CAD.

3a. Which type of neuraxial technique will you do for this patient?

I will not perform a neuraxial technique because such procedures are contraindicated in patients taking Plavix due to the risk of a neuraxial hematoma.

3b. Would you perform a neuraxial technique on a patient taking just ASA?

There is no contraindication to neuraxial technique in a patient using ASA.

Epidural in HELLP syndrome

A G1P0 presents to the labor and delivery suite in labor. She was diagnosed recently with the HELLP syndrome.

4a. Would you place an epidural in this patient?

It depends. In addition to inquiring about the routine conditions that would preclude the use of an epidural, I would also want to perform a focused history and physical to ascertain the severity of her HELLP syndrome. From the history, I would want to know how long she has had this, and whether she has noticed any easy bruising or bleeding as a result. From the physical, I will look for signs of bruising. Finally, I will look at my labs to see her platelet level and also a baseline coagulation profile.

4b. What is your cutoff regarding the platelet number in this patient prior to performing a neuraxial technique?

I do not have an absolute cutoff. Instead, I would want to trend the platelets if possible to see if they are stable or decreasing. I would also look for any signs and symptoms of thrombocytopenia.

PDHD

You are paged by the obstetric team to evaluate a 23 year old G1P1 with a post-dural puncture headache.

5a. What treatments are available for patients with PDHD?

The only definitive treatment is a blood patch, but the majority of cases of PDHD resolve on their own if left untreated. Hydration, bed rest, caffeine, Fioricet can all be given until the symptoms resolve on their own.

5b. Describe how a blood patch is performed.

A blood patch usually requires two clinicians, one to access the epidural space and the other to draw blood using sterile technique from the upper extremity. Communication between the two clinicians is of paramount importance. The first clinician accesses the epidural space as if performing an epidural anesthetic. Once the space is accessed, the second clinician uses Betadyne or an equivalent prepping solution to clean the area being used to draw blood. Using sterile gloves and equipment, the second clinician draws 20 mL of blood into a syringe and hands it to the first clinician, who then injects it through the epidural needle into the epidural space.

Neuraxial in CHF

A 75 year old male with severe congestive heart failure with an EF of 20% presents for a cystoscopy.

6a. He wishes to remain awake and asks if he could have a spinal. How do you respond?

I would not place a spinal in this patient because a spinal results in a sympathectomy, with venous pooling below the level of the spinal. As a result, there will be lower stroke volume for this patient, which will reduce his ejection fraction further and lead to cardiac compromise.

6b. Could you place an epidural?

An epidural would be a safer choice than a spinal because it allows me to slowly titrate in dilute concentrations of the anesthetic and assess the effect on the patient's cardiac status. Still, I would not want to risk compromising this patient's cardiac function further and would avoid all neuraxial techniques.

Thoracic epidural

A 55 year old female with small cell carcinoma of the lung presents for a left lower lobectomy.

7a. At what level would you place your epidural catheter for postoperative pain?

Generally the epidural is placed at the level of the incision or 1–2 levels lower.

7b. **Your resident asks you whether a spinal technique would be a better option. How do you respond?**
I would tell the resident that a spinal is not a better option over an epidural because an epidural allows for catheter placement, which will allow the titration of local anesthesia as well as narcotics during the case, thereby reducing the need for systemic anesthetics, and will also allow a conduit for administering postoperative pain relief. Additionally, a spinal anesthetic tends to be denser than an epidural and at that level could lead to difficulty in the use of muscles needed for adequate respiration and pulmonary toilet in the postoperative period.

Coumadin

You go to the ICU to remove an epidural catheter you had placed 2 days earlier on a patient for postoperative pain. Upon arrival, you learn that the surgical resident accidentally resumed this patient's coumadin dose.

8a. **How does coumadin work?**
Coumadin blocks factors 2, 7, 9, and 10 which are the vitamin K dependant coagulation factors. It also blocks protein C and S which are responsible for anticoagulation. Thus, the initial effect of coumadin is to place the patient in a procoagulant state by inhibiting factors C and S.

8b. **How could you reverse the effects of coumadin?**
Coumadin is reversed by administration of vitamin K. For emergency situations, FFP can be given to temporarily replace factors 2, 7, 9, and 10.

Asthma

You are paged to the PACU to evaluate an 18 year old patient complaining of pain after a right inguinal hernia repair under general anesthesia. She has a history of asthma and takes daily Advair.

9a. **Could you give this patient ketorolac?**
No, I would not give this patient ketorolac because she has a history of asthma. In general, patients with asthma should not receive NSAIDs because of the risk of developing an exacerbation of their asthmatic symptoms.

9b. **The patient asks you if she could have had this case performed with an epidural anesthetic. How do you respond?**
Epidural anesthesia is an option for such surgeries but the decision of whether or not to perform such a technique cannot be made unless a thorough discussion occurs with the surgeon regarding the size and dimensions of the hernia. If this were a small hernia, intense muscle relaxation was not required,

and the patient consented to the technique, then an epidural can be a good option. However, if this was a large hernia which required intense muscle relaxation and/or there were contraindications to an epidural in this patient, then I would not have entertained an epidural approach.

Spinal technique

You are supervising a first year anesthesia resident as he is performing a spinal anesthetic.

10a. Which ligaments of the back would the resident traverse in trying to reach the epidural space?
To reach the spinal canal, the resident would traverse the supraspinous, interspinous, and then the ligamentum flavum before reaching the epidural space.

10b. How does the midline approach differ from the paramedian approach?
In the midline approach, the supraspinous, interspinous, and ligamentum flavum are traversed. However, in the paramedian approach, the needle is inserted not in the midline, but 1–2 cm lateral to the spinous process, and only the ligamentum flavum is traversed.

FURTHER READING

Atchabahian A., Gupta R. (eds.) *The Anesthesia Guide*. New York: McGraw-Hill Publishing, 2013.

Barash P. G., Cullen B. F., Stoelting R. K., Cahalan M., Stock C. M. (eds.). *Clinical Anesthesia*, 6th edn. Philadelphia, PA: Lippincott Williams & Wilkins, 2009.

Horlocker T. T., Wedel D. J., Rowlingson J. C., Enneking F. K., Kopp S. L., Benzon H. T., Brown D. L., Heit J. A., Mulroy M. F., Rosenquist R. W., Tryba M., Yuan C. S. Regional anesthesia in the patient receiving antithrombotic or thrombolytic therapy. American Society of Regional Anesthesia and Pain Medicine Guidelines (Third Edition). *Reg Anesth Pain Med* 2010; 35: 64–101.

39

Critical care

Ruchir Gupta

Latex allergy

A 34 year old female presents for a laparoscopic cholecystectomy. She claims to have a severe anaphylactic allergy to latex.

1a. What precautions would you take in this patient with respect to her latex allergy?
I would take several precautions in this patient. First, I will make sure all of my anesthesia equipment (injection ports, circuit) are latex free, including the rubber stoppers on the drug vials. If there is any doubt, I will remove the stoppers and draw drugs directly from the vial. I will remove all latex rubber gloves from the OR and use nonpowdered latex-free gloves. I will make sure the OR is clearly marked as "latex free" so that all health care providers are aware throughout the case. If possible, I will try to make this the first case of the day to avoid any contamination from a previous case. Given the nature of the latex allergy, I will have my resuscitation drugs handy, including Benadryl, dexamethasone, and epinephrine, in the unlikely event this patient is exposed to latex despite these precautions. I will also have a team meeting with the surgeon and the nurses in the room to ensure they have also made the appropriate adjustments to ensure latex-free equipment is used.

1b. What medical conditions are associated with latex allergies?
Patients who have worked in the rubber industry or health care industry are at risk for latex allergy. Patients with urogenital abnormalities such as spina bifida are also at risk. Patients with an allergy to bananas and kiwi are also at risk. Finally, patients who have undergone several surgeries since childhood are also at risk.

Rapid Review Anesthesiology Oral Boards, ed. Ruchir Gupta and Minh Chau Joseph Tran. Published by Cambridge University Press. © Cambridge University Press 2013.

Hetastarch

A 36 year old female was pulled out of a burning building. She has severe burns to over 50% of her body. The patient is brought to the OR for an emergent repair of an open radius fracture.

2a. Your resident suggests you use colloid in this patient. How do you respond?

I would avoid using colloid as the primary fluid in this patient. Burn patients have leaky capillaries, which causes extravasation of proteins from the intravascular space into the extravascular compartment. Exogenous colloid administration would exacerbate this problem by worsening this outward force. Thus, I would opt to give this patient crystalloid.

2b. What are the potential side effects associated with hetastarch?

Hetastarch has several potential complications including headache, itching, parotid gland enlargement, anaphylactoid reactions, and coagulation abnormalities such as transient prolongation of prothrombin time/partial thromboplastin time and bleeding time.

Fat embolism syndrome

A 56 year old homeless male underwent an ORIF of an open right femur 2 days ago. He is now in the ICU with signs of respiratory distress.

3a. How is fat embolism syndrome diagnosed?

To diagnose fat embolism, Gurd's criteria must be employed. One sign from the major and at least four signs from the minor must be seen in order to satisfy the criteria. The major criteria are: PaO_2 <60 mmHg, axillary or subconjunctival petechiae, occurring transiently in 50–60% of cases, and CNS depression disproportionate to the hypoxemia. The minor criteria are: HR >110 bpm, temperature >38.5°C, emboli in retina, fat in urine, drop in Hct or platelets, increased ESR or plasma viscosity, and fat globules in sputum.

3b. What would you expect a chest X-ray to show in a fat embolism syndrome?

A chest X-ray routinely shows bilateral infiltrates.

Magnesium overdose

A 34 year old G1P0 with preeclampsia is receiving Mg therapy.

4a. What are the side effects of Mg?

Mg is associated with sedation, muscle weakness, cardiac depression, neonatal depression, tocolysis, prolonged labor, and respiratory depression.

4b. **What EKG abnormalities are associated with Mg overdose?**
The cardiac manifestations are different depending on the Mg level. A level between 5 and 8 mEq/L is associated with a prolongation of PR interval and widening of the QRS complex. At 15 mEq/L, one would expect sinoatrial and atrioventricular nodal block. At 25 mEq/L one would expect a full-blown cardiac arrest.

DIC

You are providing general anesthesia for a 45 year old female who is having an exploratory laparotomy for a ruptured diverticulitis. Midway through the case you notice symptoms of DIC.

5a. **How will you respond?**
DIC is a life-threatening emergency. I will call for help and immediately check the vital signs, making sure the patient is oxygenating and ventilating well on 100% O_2. I will open IV fluids wide and establish at least two large bore IV accesses (>18 g) to aid in fluid resuscitation. Next, I will administer blood products including FFP, cryoprecipitate, platelets, and PRBC through a rapid transfuser. Depending on the patient's clinical condition, I will place invasive monitors such as an arterial line and a central line to aid in the hemodynamic management of this patient.

5b. **What is DIC?**
DIC stands for disseminated intravascular coagulation. As the name implies, blood coagulates within the blood vessels, leading to a consumption of coagulation products. As a result, massive hemorrhage occurs while thrombosis ensues intravascularly. The net effect is profound anemia, hypovolemia, thrombocytopenia, and hemodynamic instability. If uncorrected, DIC leads to shock and end-organ damage.

Sarcoidosis

A 41 year old female with a history of severe sarcoidosis presents for a right knee replacement.

6a. **Would you offer a regional or general technique for this patient?**
Based on the information given, it seems likely that this patient has severe lung disease secondary to her sarcoidosis. Thus, a regional technique will allow me to avoid instrumenting the airway and instituting positive pressure ventilation. A regional technique provides superior analgesia without depressing the respiratory drive. Additionally, given her sarcoidosis, it seems likely that she will have difficulty being weaned off the ventilator.

6b. **If you did decide to conduct this case with general anesthesia, can an LMA be used?**
Yes. Depending on the length of the case, an LMA can certainly be used. Sarcoidosis does not increase the risk of aspiration. Additionally, an LMA would allow the patient to maintain spontaneous ventilation throughout the case which would minimize the amount of respiratory depressant drugs I would have to administer.

Allergic reactions

A 24 year old female presents for a left foot bunionectomy. During the administration of cefazolin, the patient develops severe hypotension, bronchospasm, and hives over her torso.

7a. **What is the mechanism of an anaphylactic reaction?**
It is mediated when the IgE antibody-antigen (cefazolin) complex binds to mast cells causing them to degranulate. The substances degranulated by mast cells and basophils lead to hypotension, bronchospasm, and ultimately full-blown cardiovascular and respiratory collapse.

7b. **How does anaphylaxis differ from anaphylactoid reactions?**
In anaphylaxis, an antigen causes the production of IgE antibodies which bind to mast cells and cause degranulation. In anaphylactoid reactions, the antigen itself binds to the mast cells and causes the degranulation.

Blood transfusion

A 44 year old Jehovah's Witness presents for a Whipple's procedure. She states she does not want a blood transfusion under any circumstances.

8a. **In what circumstances would you avoid using cell saver?**
I would avoid cell saver in conditions that lead to contamination of the surgical field with amniotic fluid, fecal material, tumor cells, Betadine, bone cement, gastric fluids, and epinephrine.

8b. **Under what circumstances would you avoid acute normovolemic hemodilution?**
I would avoid acute normovolemic hemodilution in any patient who has severe cardiac disease because anemia will cause an increase in myocardial work and increase the demand side of the supply and demand ratio. I would also avoid it in severe renal disease because the extra fluid administered to the patient would need to be effectively excreted by the kidneys. The patient will not be able to get rid of the excess fluid and may develop CHF and electrolyte abnormalities. Finally, I would avoid it in conditions where the patient's baseline Hb is already low (<11 g/dL).

Aspiration

You are performing general anesthesia with an LMA on a 63 year old patient who is having a right knee arthroscopy.

9a. Mid way through the case, you notice the patient is coughing and her oropharynx is filled with the Bicitra you gave her preoperatively for her GERD. How do you respond?

I would immediately remove the LMA, suction the oropharynx, put the back of the head up, and emergently intubate the patient. I would ventilate with 100% O_2, and auscultate the chest for any abnormal breath sounds. I would add PEEP to my ventilator and administer a beta-agonist nebulizer as needed. I will assess the BP and heart rate and consider opening the fluids wide and treating the hypotension with a pressor. Finally, I will ask for a chest X-ray to be done in the PACU.

9b. The case continues uneventfully and the patient is easily extubated. Will you discharge this patient home as planned or admit her for an overnight stay at the hospital?

It depends on the course of her surgery. If the patient continued to show no signs of respiratory distress for 2 hours in the PACU and her breath sounds were clear to auscultation with a normal appearing chest X-ray, I would allow her to be discharged with follow-up to her medical doctor. If, however, she was desaturating in the PACU and/or had wheezing and needed beta-agonist therapy, then I would admit her for overnight stay and consider consulting the pulmonary service.

TPN

A 64 year old homeless male was found unresponsive by the emergency medical services. He is currently in the ICU and is receiving TPN via a central line.

10a. What is refeeding syndrome?

Refeeding syndrome is a syndrome of electrolyte imbalances that is seen when a patient receives TPN therapy after a period of starvation. Patients with anorexia, kwashiorkor, marasmus, and chronic alcoholism are at greatest risk. The electrolyte abnormalities most commonly seen are hypophosphatemia, hypokalemia, hypomagnesemia, glucose imbalance, vitamin deficiency, and fluid imbalance.

10b. What other complications of TPN would you be wary of?

TPN therapy is associated with bacterial infection, fatty liver, venous thrombosis, metabolic acidosis, and hypercarbia.

FURTHER READING

Atchabahian A., Gupta R. (eds.). *The Anesthesia Guide*. New York: McGraw Hill Publishing, 2013.

Miller R. D., Eriksson L. I., Fleisher L. A., Wiener-Kornish J. P., Young W. L. (eds.). *Miller's Anesthesia*, 7th edn. Philadelphia, PA: Churchill Livingstone Elsevier, 2010.

Algorithm appendix

1. ASA difficult airway

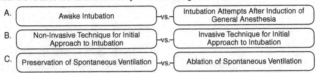

AMERICAN SOCIETY OF ANESTHESIOLOGISTS

DIFFICULT AIRWAY ALGORITHM

1. Assess the likelihood and clinical impact of basic management problems:
   - A. Difficult Ventilation
   - B. Difficult Intubation
   - C. Difficulty with Patient Cooperation or Consent
   - D. Difficult Tracheostomy

2. Actively pursue opportunities to deliver supplemental oxygen throughout the process of difficult airway management

3. Consider the relative merits and feasibility of basic management choices:

A. Awake Intubation –vs.– Intubation Attempts After Induction of General Anesthesia

B. Non-Invasive Technique for Initial Approach to Intubation –vs.– Invasive Technique for Initial Approach to Intubation

C. Preservation of Spontaneous Ventilation –vs.– Ablation of Spontaneous Ventilation

4. Develop primary and alternative strategies:

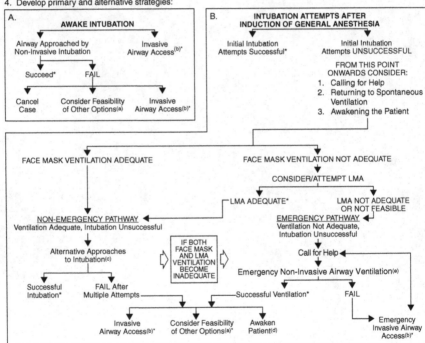

* Confirm ventilation, tracheal intubation, or LMA placement with exhaled CO_2

a. Other options include (but are not limited to): surgery utilizing face mask or LMA anesthesia, local anesthesia infiltration or regional nerve blockade. Pursuit of these options usually implies that mask ventilation will not be problematic. Therefore, these options may be of limited value if this step in the algorithm has been reached via the Emergency Pathway.

b. Invasive airway access includes surgical or percutaneous tracheostomy or cricothyrotomy.

c. Alternative non-invasive approaches to difficult intubation include (but are not limited to): use of different laryngoscope blades, LMA as an intubation conduit (with or without fiberoptic guidance), fiberoptic intubation, intubating stylet or tube changer, light wand, retrograde intubation, and blind oral or nasal intubation.

d. Consider re-preparation of the patient for awake intubation or canceling surgery.

e. Options for emergency non-invasive airway ventilation include (but are not limited to): rigid bronchoscope, esophageal-tracheal combitube ventilation, or transtracheal jet ventilation.

2.   Fire in the OR algorithm

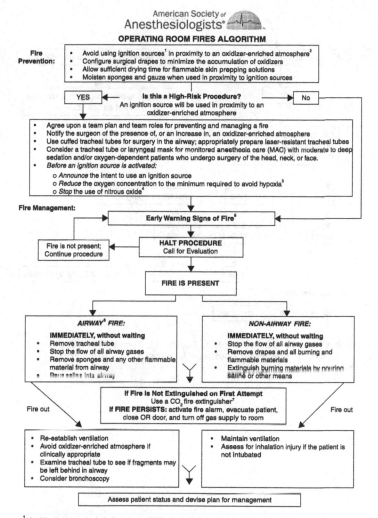

American Society of
Anesthesiologists®
OPERATING ROOM FIRES ALGORITHM

Fire Prevention:
- Avoid using ignition sources[1] in proximity to an oxidizer-enriched atmosphere[2]
- Configure surgical drapes to minimize the accumulation of oxidizers
- Allow sufficient drying time for flammable skin prepping solutions
- Moisten sponges and gauze when used in proximity to ignition sources

Is this a High-Risk Procedure?
An ignition source will be used in proximity to an oxidizer-enriched atmosphere

→ YES

→ No

- Agree upon a team plan and team roles for preventing and managing a fire
- Notify the surgeon of the presence of, or an increase in, an oxidizer-enriched atmosphere
- Use cuffed tracheal tubes for surgery in the airway; appropriately prepare laser-resistant tracheal tubes
- Consider a tracheal tube or laryngeal mask for monitored anesthesia care (MAC) with moderate to deep sedation and/or oxygen-dependent patients who undergo surgery of the head, neck, or face.
- *Before an ignition source is activated:*
  o *Announce* the intent to use an ignition source
  o *Reduce* the oxygen concentration to the minimum required to avoid hypoxia[3]
  o *Stop* the use of nitrous oxide[4]

Fire Management:

Early Warning Signs of Fire[5]

Fire is not present; Continue procedure ←

HALT PROCEDURE
Call for Evaluation

FIRE IS PRESENT

AIRWAY[6] FIRE:

IMMEDIATELY, without waiting
- Remove tracheal tube
- Stop the flow of all airway gases
- Remove sponges and any other flammable material from airway
- Pour saline into airway

NON-AIRWAY FIRE:

IMMEDIATELY, without waiting
- Stop the flow of all airway gases
- Remove drapes and all burning and flammable materials
- Extinguish burning materials by pouring saline or other means

If Fire is Not Extinguished on First Attempt
Use a CO_2 fire extinguisher[7]
If FIRE PERSISTS: activate fire alarm, evacuate patient, close OR door, and turn off gas supply to room

Fire out

Fire out

- Re-establish ventilation
- Avoid oxidizer-enriched atmosphere if clinically appropriate
- Examine tracheal tube to see if fragments may be left behind in airway
- Consider bronchoscopy

- Maintain ventilation
- Assess for inhalation injury if the patient is not intubated

Assess patient status and devise plan for management

[1] Ignition sources include but are not limited to electrosurgery or electrocautery units and lasers.

[2] An oxidizer-enriched atmosphere occurs when there is any increase in oxygen concentration above room air level, and/or the pressure of any concentration of nitrous oxide.

[3] After minimizing delivered oxygen, wait a period of time ((*e.g.*, 1-3 min) before using an ignition source. For oxygen dependent patients, reduce supplemental oxygen delivery to the minimum required to avoid hypoxia. Monitor oxygenation with pulse oximetry, and if feasible, inspired, exhaled, and/or delivered oxygen concentration.

[4] After stopping the delivery of nitrous oxide, wait a period of time (*e.g.*, 1-3 min) before using an ignition source.

[5] Unexpected flash, flame, smoke or heat, unusual sounds ((*e.g.*, a "pop," snap or "foomp") or odors, unexpected movement of drapes, discoloration of drapes or breathing circuit, unexpected patient movement or complaint.

[6] In this algorithm, airway fire refers to a fire in the airway or breathing circuit.

[7] A CO_2 fire extinguisher may be used on the patient if necessary.

3.   Bare metal stent and anticoagulation management algorithm

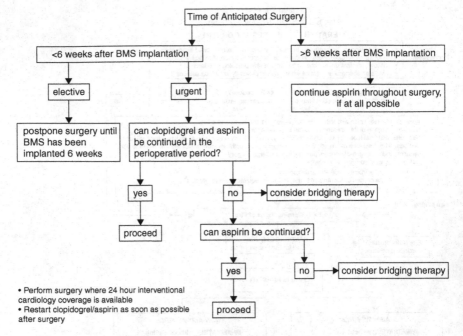

- Perform surgery where 24 hour interventional cardiology coverage is available
- Restart clopidogrel/aspirin as soon as possible after surgery

*Newsome L.T., Weller R.S., Gernancher J.C., Kutcher M.A., Royster R.L. Coronary Artery Stents: II. Perioperative Considerations and management. Anesthesia & Analgesia 2008; 107(2):570-590. Reproduced with permission.

4. Drug eluting stent and anticoagulation management algorithm

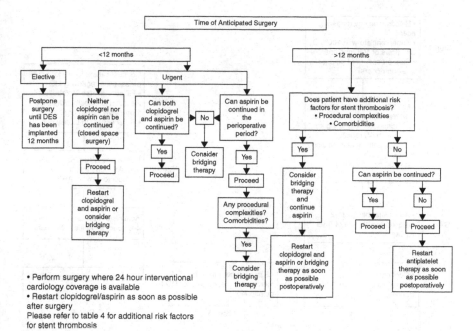

• Perform surgery where 24 hour interventional cardiology coverage is available
• Restart clopidogrel/aspirin as soon as possible after surgery
Please refer to table 4 for additional risk factors for stent thrombosis

*Newsome L.T., Weller R.S., Gernancher J.C., Kutcher M.A., Royster R.L. Coronary Artery Stents: II. Perioperative Considerations and management. Anesthesia & Analgesia 2008; 107(2):570-590. Reproduced with permission.

5.   Malignant hyperthermia algorithm

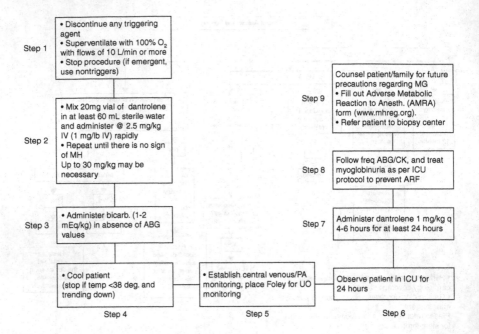

Step 1
• Discontinue any triggering agent
• Superventilate with 100% O_2 with flows of 10 L/min or more
• Stop procedure (if emergent, use nontriggers)

Step 2
• Mix 20mg vial of dantrolene in at least 60 mL sterile water and administer @ 2.5 mg/kg IV (1 mg/lb IV) rapidly
• Repeat until there is no sign of MH
Up to 30 mg/kg may be necessary

Step 3
• Administer bicarb. (1-2 mEq/kg) in absence of ABG values

Step 4
• Cool patient
(stop if temp <38 deg. and trending down)

Step 5
• Establish central venous/PA monitoring, place Foley for UO monitoring

Step 6
Observe patient in ICU for 24 hours

Step 7
Administer dantrolene 1 mg/kg q 4-6 hours for at least 24 hours

Step 8
Follow freq ABG/CK, and treat myoglobinuria as per ICU protocol to prevent ARF

Step 9
Counsel patient/family for future precautions regarding MG
• Fill out Adverse Metabolic Reaction to Anesth. (AMRA) form (www.mhreg.org).
• Refer patient to biopsy center

Index

Printed in the United States
By Bookmasters